30p

PLATINUM VIGNETTES™

ULTRA-HIGH-YIELD CLINICAL CASE SCENARIOS
FOR USMLE STEP 2

Psychiatry

PLATINUM VIGNETTES™

ULTRA-HIGH-YIELD CLINICAL CASE SCENARIOS FOR USMLE STEP 2

Psychiatry

ADAM BROCHERT, MD

Resident
Department of Radiology
Medical College of Georgia
Memorial Health University Medical Center
Savannah, Georgia

Hanley & Belfus, Inc. / Philadelphia

Publisher: HANLEY & BELFUS, INC.
Medical Publishers
210 South 13th Street
Philadelphia, PA 19107
(215) 546-7293; 800-962-1892
FAX (215) 790-9330
Web site: http://www.hanleyandbelfus.com

Note to the reader: Although the information in this book has been carefully reviewed for correctness of dosage and indications, neither the author nor the publisher can accept any legal responsibility for any errors or omissions that may be made. Neither the publisher nor the author makes any warranty, expressed or implied, with respect to the material contained herein. Before prescribing any drug, the reader must review the manufacturer's current product information (package inserts) for accepted indications, absolute dosage recommendations, and other information pertinent to the safe and effective use of the product described. This is especially important when drugs are given in combination or as an adjunct to other forms of therapy.

PLATINUM VIGNETTES™: PSYCHIATRY ISBN 1-56053-534-2

Library of Congress Control Number: 2002102759

Last digit is the print number: 9 8 7 6 5 4 3 2 1

INTRODUCTION

Case scenarios are a great way to review for the USMLE Step 2 exam. A high percentage of current exam questions center on case studies or patient presentations in an office or emergency department setting. Practicing this format and being familiar with the majority of the classic, "guaranteed-to-be-on-the-exam" case scenarios gives the examinee an obvious, clear-cut advantage. *Platinum Vignettes*™ were written to offer you that advantage.

You need to be familiar not only with pathophysiology, but also the work-up and management of several conditions to succeed on the USMLE Step 2 exam. Sifting through the history, physical exam findings, and various tests, you are expected to make and confirm the diagnosis and manage the patient's condition.

Each book in the *Platinum Vignettes*™ presents 50 case scenarios or clinical vignettes. The individual vignettes are followed by the diagnosis, pathophysiology, diagnostic strategies, and management issues pertaining to that specific patient. The reader must turn the page to obtain these latter details, and is encouraged to "guess" before reading about the patient's condition and course. In fact, you are advised not only to guess the diagnosis, but also to postulate on which test to order next, what therapy to give, and what to "watch out" for in the condition presented.

Important words or phrases ("buzzwords") are set in bold type in the explanation of each vignette. These words or phrases indicate the material most commonly asked about on the exam or are important in helping to distinguish one condition from another. This format is designed for review of material that was previously learned during rotations; therefore, further reading is advised if the topic or buzzwords are unfamiliar. Remember, buzzwords are rarely helpful unless you know what they mean!

Every attempt was made to provide the most current, up-to-date information on every topic tackled in this volume and every volume in the series—but medicine is a rapidly changing field. If you hear about a new therapy in a conference or on rounds, it may well be that the standard of care has changed. Remember, though, that what you see on the wards and in the office isn't always applicable to the boards (e.g., everyone with pneumonia should not be given the latest "big-gun" antibiotic; all patients with headaches should not receive a CT scan).

Good luck!

ADAM BROCHERT, MD

NOTE: A standard Table of Contents, with cases listed by diagnosis, would give you too much of a head start on solving each patient scenario. Challenge yourself! When ready, you can turn to the detailed Case Index at the back of this book.

Child Psychiatry

History

A mother brings in her 11-year-old son because she discovered him and a male friend of the same age in the basement with their pants down. The boys were staring at each other's genitalia when she walked into the room. She wants you to tell her if her son is homosexual, and if so, what treatment is available. The boy is clearly embarrassed and avoids eye contact with you while his mother is talking. The mother states that her son has never done anything like this before as far as she knows and otherwise seems "perfectly normal." He is a good student and is involved in athletics at school. He has no medical problems and takes no medications. The mother reports that he has many friends, primarily male.

Interview/Exam

You ask the mother to leave the room, and the boy is clearly uncomfortable. He answers questions appropriately and seems alert, oriented, and intelligent. His mood and affect appear normal, and he looks healthy. He denies ever engaging in similar types of behavior in the past. The boy claims that he is a virgin and is not interested in sexual relations with either sex. He denies having any sexual impulses.

Tests

None

Pathophysiology

Psychiatry and pediatrics are common areas for board examiners to present you with a **normal situation** or presentation to try to trick you into calling it abnormal or treating something that shouldn't be treated. Sexual experimentation—both heterosexual and homosexual—is *normal* at this age. One well-known investigator (Kinsey) collected data suggesting that almost **half of prepubertal males** have some type of genital experience with another male peer. If the boy turns out to be homosexual, this is a normal variant, not a disorder. **Treatment is not indicated for homosexuality,** nor is it effective if attempted.

Diagnosis & Treatment

There is a wide range of what is considered normal in sexuality. Occasional **cross-dressing, fetishism, voyeurism, sadism/masochism,** and **viewing of pornography** are all examples of **normal variations** in sexual behavior. Be careful not to label these behaviors as pathologic on the boards (regardless of your personal or moral opinion).

When activities are excessive and/or interfere with normal functioning, or when arousal is not possible in the absence of the activity, situation, or inanimate object, a disorder may be present.

In children—especially younger children—recurrent sexual "play" may be a marker for **sexual abuse.** On Step 2, watch for other findings in this setting that suggest such abuse (e.g., problems in school, trauma to the genitalia).

More High-Yield Facts

Homosexuality is thought to be due to a combination of **genetics and environment.** Approximately **2–5% of adults** are exclusively homosexual, though a much larger percentage have experimented with homosexual sex. Most homosexuals (just like heterosexuals) begin to notice their sexual preference in **early adolescence;** however, clear recognition of sexual orientation often does not begin until late adolescence or early adulthood.

Child Psychiatry

History

You are seeing a 6-year-old girl because over the past month she has almost always refused to go to school. The child told her parents that she cannot go to school because her mother may get kidnapped while she is gone. Despite numerous attempts to motivate, reassure, and even bribe the child with candy and toys, she still refuses to go to school on most days. The child also seems to resort to sudden stomachaches in the morning before school to avoid having to go, according to the mother.

At one point, the parents became frustrated and dropped their daughter off at school against her wishes. They received a call 30 minutes later from the child's teacher because the child was crying and hysterical, and the parents had to go pick her up. Similar behavior occurs if the parents try to leave the child with a babysitter. The child is otherwise healthy, has no significant past medical history, and takes no medications. There are no physical symptoms according to the mother, other than the stomachaches. Symptoms are entirely absent when either parent is around the child, and there is no threat of separation.

Interview/Exam

Height and weight are normal for age, and the patient appears healthy. Upon questioning, she admits fearing that her mother will be kidnapped by "people wearing masks" if she goes to school or is otherwise separated from her mother. She doesn't worry about her dad, because he can "beat up" the kidnappers. The child is alert and seems intelligent.

Tests

None

Pathophysiology

Separation anxiety is very common in **school-age children,** but often can be overcome. A formal disorder is diagnosed when there is **excessive** and **inappropriate** anxiety. **Depression** typically coexists. Separation anxiety can be **learned or inherited,** and an **overprotective or fearful parent** may increase the risk of this disorder. **External life stressors** play a role in some children.

Diagnosis & Treatment

As with any psychiatric disorder, it is important to rule out an organic cause. Hyperthyroidism, hyperadrenalism, and pheochromocytoma are potential etiologies of anxiety (though extremely unlikely in the case presented, given the absence of symptoms during parent contact). Historically, a **move, parental death or illness, new school,** or other change in the child's environment precipitates symptoms.

To make the diagnosis, the child must have inappropriate and excessive anxiety concerning **separation from the home or from parents/caretakers.** This may be manifested by excessive distress when separation occurs or is anticipated, **worry about harm to or loss of the parents** (including nightmares about the child getting lost or the parent being kidnapped), **refusal to go to school** or elsewhere due to fear of separation, and **fear of being alone or going to sleep without attachment figures. Physical (somatic) complaints** are also classic, such as **headaches, stomachaches,** and **nausea.** These mysteriously appear at just the right time and go away once the threat of separation ceases. As with all psychiatric disorders, the symptoms must impair functioning or cause significant distress and cannot be due to another condition.

Initial treatment involves **psychotherapy,** often in the form of **cognitive-behavioral therapy.** This is one of the most effective treatments. Systematic desensitization and other behavioral techniques may be effective. **Antidepressants** may be used as adjunctive therapy in severe cases that fail non-pharmacologic management or if depression coexists. (Selective serotonin-reuptake inhibitors such as fluoxetine are preferred over tricyclics.) Benzodiazepines and/or inpatient treatment on a short-term basis may be needed for the most severe cases.

More High-Yield Facts

Most cases begin between **5 and 12 years of age,** and symptoms must begin *prior to 18* for the diagnosis to be made. Additionally, symptoms must have been present for at least 4 weeks.

Case 3

Child Psychiatry

History

Your patient is an 8-year-old boy who is quite disruptive both at home and at school. In fact, one of his teachers recommended a psychiatric consultation for disruptive classroom behavior. The teacher has complained that the child is disobedient and inattentive, often disrupting the class and disturbing and distracting the other children. The mother states that her son "always seems to be going 100 miles per minute, ever since he was 2 years old." The boy is usually restless and has trouble paying attention, and becomes frustrated and even hostile when asked to do chores that require concentration, such as homework.

The child also displays unusual risk-taking behavior, apparently without stopping to consider consequences. For example, he crosses the street suddenly and without looking, even after being repeatedly scolded and taught how to look both ways before crossing. The mother reports that the child has few close friends.

Interview/Exam

The patient fidgets throughout the interview and has trouble paying attention; he frequently interrupts with questions about the room décor and other subjects. His concentration is impaired, seemingly because of a shortened attention span, though he seems to have normal intelligence. Height and weight are normal for age.

Tests

None

Pathophysiology

ADHD is estimated to affect roughly 3.5 million children, about **3–5%** of children in the U.S. **Males are affected more often** than females by a ratio of approximately 4:1. The disorder begins **before the age of 7 years** (by definition), but may last into adulthood. There appears to be some **genetic basis,** as infants can be affected, and incidence is increased in siblings of those with ADHD. In addition, there is an increased incidence of **alcoholism** and antisocial personality disorder in affected children's parents. (ADHD risk may be increased in kids whose mothers drank alcohol during pregnancy.)

Diagnosis & Treatment

Again, as with any psychiatric disorder, you must rule out an organic cause, even though most children will have a lifelong history of ADHD. **Head trauma** can cause impulsivity and concentration problems, and some cases may be attributable to in **utero insult** (e.g., **alcohol,** infections). Symptoms start at an early age (often by 3 years old), but typically are not brought to clinical attention until a child **begins school.** Duration of symptoms must be at least 6 months; symptoms must not be due to another disorder; and they must cause significant impairment in **multiple settings** (e.g., home and school).

The diagnosis is made by history and examination. The hallmarks of the disorder are **inattention, hyperactivity,** and **impulsivity.** Memorizing and understanding these three classes of symptoms in common-sense terms will suffice for the Step 2 exam (the DSM-IV specific criteria are somewhat extensive). **Learning disabilities** are characteristic (70%, usually mild) and must be addressed. **Developmental delays, coordination problems, poor social skills,** and **low self-esteem** are common comorbidities.

Treatment is **stimulants,** usually the **amphetamine** class (e.g., **methylphenidate,** dextroamphetamine, or pemoline), along with psychotherapy. **Antidepressants** may help in some, as coexisting **depression and/or anxiety** are also common.

More High-Yield Facts

Amphetamine side-effects are high yield: **growth suppression** (monitor growth during therapy, and use drug holidays during school vacations to allow rebound growth), **insomnia, abdominal pain, anorexia,** and addiction. The use of amphetamines occasionally unmasks a **tic disorder** (e.g., Tourette's), which is noted in up to 20% of those with ADHD.

Child Psychiatry

History

A father brings in his 9-year-old son because of concern about physical behaviors that began over a year ago, but have become more frequent, now occurring several times a day. The behaviors include repetitive eye blinking and facial grimacing, and the boy also seems to clear his throat every few minutes. A recent development is grunting—which is upsetting to the child and prompted today's visit.

The patient's father reports that he is a "good kid" who does well in school and has several friends. The boy does not cause trouble at home or school and has a good appetite and an upbeat mood most of the time.

Interview/Exam

The patient appears healthy and alert, though he is easily distracted. He is intelligent and appropriate. During the interview, you observe multiple sudden, rapid, and non-rhythmic episodes of eye-blinking and facial grimacing, which are seemingly involuntary. The child also occasionally grunts during the interview when not talking, which seems to frustrate him. Height and weight are normal for age.

Tests

None

Pathophysiology

TD is now thought to be an **organic/neurologic disorder,** rather than functional/psychiatric. A **genetic basis** is suspected, as evidenced by increased concordance rates in twin studies and increased risk in relatives of those affected. Some believe that the disorder is transmitted in an **autosomal dominant** fashion with variable penetrance and expression, and **genetic imprinting** may play a role, as sons of mothers with TD seem to have even greater risk. **Males are affected more often** than females by a ratio of roughly 3:1. The overall prevalence is about **1 in 2000,** though minor tic disorders are more common.

Diagnosis & Treatment

Symptoms must last at least 1 year, begin **prior to 18 years of age,** and cause impairment or distress. Symptoms usually first start around **6–9 years of age.** The hallmark of TD is **tics,** which are **involuntary, sudden, rapid, repetitive, purposeless, nonrhythmic, and stereotyped actions.** In Tourette's, both vocal and motor tics must be present, though not necessarily at the same time. Common motor tics include **eye blinking, facial grimacing, head or neck shaking/jerking, and lip smacking.** Common vocal tics include **throat clearing, grunting, barking, hissing, humming,** or the classic **coprolalia** (uttering obscenities, seen in one-third of cases). Tics usually occur on a **daily basis** and may worsen with **stress or fatigue.**

Up to 50% of those with TD have attention-deficit hyperactivity disorder **(ADHD),** and treatment of ADHD with **stimulants may unmask** an underlying TD or tic disorder. This is a classic atypical presentation, occurring in up to 25% of diagnosed cases. If a child treated with stimulants develops new-onset of tics during therapy, strongly consider **stopping the drug** (must weigh risks/benefits). Obsessive-compulsive symptoms are also common in affected children. Tourette's tends to be a **chronic, lifelong disorder** with **exacerbations and remissions.** Severe symptoms can result in **social isolation** and secondary **depression.**

Treatment is **supportive** in mild cases with minimal functional impairment. **Clonidine** or **antipsychotics** (usually haloperidol or pimozide) are often effective for more severe symptoms. Psychotherapy rarely helps treat the disorder, but may help patients accept and adjust to it.

More High-Yield Facts

Seizures or **chorea** (e.g., rheumatic fever) are differential considerations. History/lack of other symptoms rules out rheumatic fever. Seizures (but not TD) usually cause **impaired consciousness** during involuntary movement.

Child Psychiatry

History

A 15-year-old girl has made an appointment at the insistence of her mother. The mother is very concerned because she found her daughter intentionally inducing herself to vomit last week. The mother mentions that her daughter has strange eating habits, often not eating for several days. The patient is an average student and has few friends, which the mother feels is due to low self-esteem.

Interview/Exam

The patient appears well developed and well nourished; cursory examination reveals normal sexual development. She is slightly overweight. You note excoriations on the skin overlying her knuckles, as well as some asymmetric enamel erosion on the posterior aspect of several teeth. She denies any menstrual irregularities.

The patient is alert, oriented, and appropriate. She does not seem depressed. When asked about her behavior, she admits to inducing vomiting to keep her weight down. This behavior began roughly 2 years ago when her parents divorced and has become more and more frequent. She also mentions episodes of eating large quantities of food roughly three times a week, usually late at night when no one can see her, separated by periods of disinterest in food. During the eating episodes, the patient reports a sensation of losing control and inability to stop eating until she experiences physical pain. She says that she is not sexually active primarily because she is overweight and unattractive. The patient denies depression, but admits to feeling worthless and disgusted with herself for a brief period after one of her eating episodes.

Tests

None

Pathophysiology

Bulimia is a common eating disorder that affects **up to 40% of college women** at some point. It is more common than anorexia and has a **better prognosis.** Both anorexia and bulimia stem partly from a **distorted sense of body image** and **societal pressures** to be thin. Both eating disorders are quite rare in countries where food is scarce. **Females are much more commonly affected** than males (by a 10–20:1 ratio)

Diagnosis & Treatment

Bulimia usually begins in **mid to late adolescence** and is classic in women attending college. The hallmarks of the disorder are **"binging"** (binge-eating) and **"purging."** *Binging* refers to **consumption of large amounts of food over a brief period of time,** stemming from **uncontrollable impulses** to eat that may only be satisfied in some patients by feeling physically ill from overeating. Patients feel a **lack of control over eating behavior** during the binges. *Purging* refers to attempts to **prevent weight gain** and/or reverse the effects of the binging episodes by **inducing vomiting, using laxatives/diuretics, dieting/fasting,** and/or **engaging in vigorous exercise.** To make the diagnosis, these episodes must occur at least twice a week for 3 months.

The self-evaluations of bulimic (and anorexic) patients are overly influenced by their perceptions of their body shape and weight. Those with bulimia are **often of normal weight and may even be slightly overweight,** and menstruation is not generally affected (differential points compared to anorexia). Binging and purging causes weight **fluctuations** over time. Classic physical findings include **excoriations of the skin over the knuckles** (from sticking the fingers down the throat) and **enamel erosion of the posterior aspects of the teeth or dental caries** (from effects of stomach acid on the teeth). **Esophagitis, electrolyte disturbances, and dehydration** can occur in more severe cases.

Treatment is difficult, but centers around **psychotherapy,** including **cognitive/ behavioral** methods and **group therapy. Antidepressants** may help. Hospitalization may be required in severe cases, such as when electrolyte disturbances or dehydration occurs. **Anorexia and bulimia commonly coexist (25–50% of cases).**

More High-Yield Facts

A higher incidence of **substance abuse** (30%, likely related to impulsivity), **affective disorders** (especially depression), and **borderline personality disorder** is noted in those affected by bulimia.

Child Psychiatry

History

A 13-year-old boy has been forced to come see you by his school's principal for repeated acts of misconduct, including a recent episode in which the patient pulled a knife on one of his teachers. The patient's mother says she has "given up hope" and thinks their coming to see you is a "waste of time," as he has been a difficult child since early grade school. She says the boy takes after his father, an abusive alcoholic who left shortly after the patient was born.

She reports that the boy frequently skips school and has been arrested three times on charges of stealing, vandalism, and setting fire to a neighbor's dog. She has caught her son drinking and smoking marijuana on multiple occasions.

Interview/Exam

The patient smiles and even giggles a few times during your conversation with his mother. He looks physically healthy, though somewhat unkempt. He says he is "a pretty good kid" who "doesn't need a shrink." The patient seems fairly intelligent and even charming at times, and is alert and oriented. When asked about the knife-pulling incident at school, he becomes sullen and refuses to talk about it, mentioning only that his teacher is "lucky" she didn't get stabbed. The boy then refuses to talk any further and simply stares at the wall and fidgets during the rest of the interview, ignoring all remaining questions.

Tests

None

Pathophysiology

Conduct disorder is the **pediatric equivalent of antisocial personality disorder.** The etiology is thought to be part genetic and part environmental, as many children with the disorder have parents who are either antisocial or alcoholics, and chaotic home/family situations are the norm. **Males are affected much more commonly** than females, by at least a 4:1 ratio.

Diagnosis & Treatment

Patients have a **poorly formed or absent conscience** and are constantly **breaking rules/laws** and **violating the rights of others. Stealing, lying, running away, setting fires, skipping school, physical cruelty** to other people and to animals, **rape, fighting, vandalism,** and **"conning" others** are all classic (also DSM-IV diagnostic criteria). **Lack of remorse, narcissism, anger,** and **low tolerance for frustration** are all usually present to some degree, and **drug/alcohol abuse** is quite common. The pattern of behavior is generally long-standing (though it may not start until adolescence) and must begin **before age 18.**

Look for **antisocial personality disorder** and/or **addictions** *in the parents,* as well as a **home life** featuring abuse, negligence, lack of discipline, and low socioeconomic status. Attention-deficit hyperactivity disorder often coexists.

Treatment is very difficult, as patients typically are not interested, and the family often cannot or will not participate in therapy. Consider removing the patient from the home in severe cases. **Psychotherapy** is generally employed, and is most effective when started at a young age. **Medications usually are not effective,** except to treat coexisting problems (e.g., hyperactivity, depression), but antipsychotics and mood stabilizers (e.g., lithium, valproic acid) can help curb violent behavior.

More High-Yield Facts

Oppositional defiant disorder (ODD) is somewhat similar to conduct disorder in that patients are hostile, negative, and defiant when interacting with adults. However, kids with ODD are *not* cruel, lying criminals ("con artists") without a conscience, who violate the rights of others. They often have behavioral problems in one or two settings (e.g., home, school), but fairly normal behavior elsewhere (e.g., during the psychiatric interview, when with peers). Conduct disorder patients display abnormal, destructive behavior in *any* setting.

Case 7

Child Psychiatry

History

A father brings in his 9-year-old daughter for evaluation. He says that he has found her walking aimlessly in the hallway at night while apparently asleep. This has happened three different times, and he wonders if she needs treatment. During each episode, the child gave incoherent responses when asked questions, and the father simply redirected her back to bed. According to the father, the child had no recollection of any of these events and has never hurt herself during the episodes. She is otherwise healthy, is a good student, and has no other medical problems. She takes no regular medications. The dad says that his ex-wife's parents used to talk about her childhood sleepwalking, but the father never noticed this behavior in his ex-wife while they were married.

Interview/Exam

The patient seems to be a happy, well-adjusted child of normal height and weight for her age. She is alert and appropriate. When asked about the incidents, she denies any knowledge of them. She claims to sleep well, and denies bedwetting or recent nightmares.

Tests

None

Pathophysiology

Sleepwalking is **common:** 15–30% of children ages 6–12 have at least one episode. A genetic influence is felt to be partly responsible, as **up to 80% of those affected have a family history of sleepwalking,** and it may be related to a mild neurologic abnormality. Episodes generally occur during **sleep stages 3 and 4** (deep, non-REM sleep).

Diagnosis & Treatment

A sleepwalking episode is characterized by **rising from bed during sleep and walking about,** usually in the **first one-third of the night.** While sleepwalking, people have a **blank, staring face and are relatively unresponsive** to the attempts of others to communicate with them. Sleepwalkers can only be awakened with **great difficulty** and generally **respond incoherently** if at all when spoken to.

Behaviors exhibited during sleepwalking can include sitting up in bed, getting dressed, using the bathroom, and talking, as well as more **dangerous activities** such as walking outside and driving (adults). Upon awakening (either from the sleepwalking or the next morning), the person generally has **amnesia for the episode.** If awakened during an episode, he or she may suffer a **short period of confusion or disorientation,** which is why many recommend *avoiding* vigorous attempts to wake the sleepwalker. Within a few minutes, any impairment of mental activity or behavior disappears—an important fact that distinguishes sleepwalking from **seizure disorder,** which can (rarely) mimic sleepwalking (but often features a significant post-ictal state).

Sleepwalking is generally considered normal (as in this case), and **rarely qualifies as a disorder.** Episodes must be **recurrent** and cause **significant distress or impairment** in functioning to be considered a disorder. Treatment is usually **conservative,** and gentle redirection back to bed may be all that is needed. Symptoms **often remit by adolescence,** but some are affected into adulthood. Consider treatment, such as locks for bedroom doors and windows and medications, for patients who engage in dangerous behaviors while sleepwalking. **Benzodiazepines** (which decrease stage 3 and 4 sleep) and sedating antidepressants may help reduce the number of episodes in severe cases.

More High-Yield Facts

Medications, such as tranquilizers or sleeping pills, may occasionally *cause or exacerbate* sleepwalking. **Stress** and extreme **tiredness**/sleep deprivation may also exacerbate attacks.

Case 8

Child Psychiatry

History

A 5-year-old girl has been referred by her family physician for continued complaints of abdominal pain in the absence of an identifiable organic cause. The work-up was extensive, and the referring doctor now wonders if there may be a functional component to the abdominal pain. Chart review reveals a history of three urinary tract infections (UTIs) in the last 18 months, but a work-up for congenital urinary tract abnormalities was negative. The child has also dropped to below the 5th percentile for weight and height in her age group, though previously, she was near the 50th percentile. Extensive endocrine work-up was negative.

The mother says her daughter has been fairly withdrawn over the last year or so and doesn't seem to be her usual happy self. The mother works full-time while her second husband (the child's stepfather), who she says has "a drinking problem," stays home and watches the child. They have been married for 1.5 years.

Interview/Exam

The patient is shy and anxious, not wanting to leave her mother's side and avoiding any eye contact. A physical exam reveals no abdominal tenderness to deep palpation and normal bowel sounds. You note a bruise on the child's inner, upper thigh. When you ask her where the bruise came from, she begins to cry. You ask the mother to remove the child's underpants to perform a genital exam and the child begins to kick and scream violently. You are unable to perform the exam. The remainder of the exam is normal, and the child calms down immediately once you begin to examine other body parts.

Tests

None

Pathophysiology

The sexual abuse of children is much more common than previously thought. It is estimated that **150,000–200,000 new cases** occur each year. Risk factors include a **child living in a single-parent home, marital conflict, a history of sexual or physical abuse perpetrated by or against the parents, and parental substance abuse.** Abuse is most commonly perpetrated by **males against females,** but other combinations do occur. The offender is **usually well-known to the child,** and often a **respected authority figure or family member** (e.g., parent, uncle, older sibling, family friend, caretaker). The peak age range of sexually abused children is **9–12,** though 25% of cases occur in children less than 8 years old.

Diagnosis & Treatment

There are no consistent symptoms of sexual abuse. **Failure to thrive, repeated UTIs, difficulty in walking or sitting, genital or rectal discharge, bruising, itching, pain, and/or bleeding** raises the possibility of sexual or other physical abuse. Very young children who seem to have explicit sexual knowledge or engage in excessive sexual play with peers have often been abused. The child may be **withdrawn and/or aggressive,** and low self-esteem and mistrust of adults are typical. **Vague abdominal pain** is a classic complaint in those who are abused. Note that signs of nonsexual physical abuse or neglect should prompt a thorough examination to look for evidence of sexual abuse. Evidence of genital trauma or rectal or genital discharge is sexual abuse *"until proven otherwise"* (a slam dunk on the boards).

Suspected sexual abuse must be reported immediately. Proof is *not* needed, and a doctor *cannot be sued* for reporting a suspicion of abuse. If necessary, the child should be **admitted to the hospital and/or placed in protective custody;** local child protective services should be notified. Obtain an x-ray **skeletal bone survey** ("child abuse survey") to seek other evidence of abuse (i.e., healing fractures). Treatment involves **psychotherapy,** both for the child and the family/perpetrator. Medications may be useful to treat associated problems (e.g., depression).

More High-Yield Facts

Childhood abuse markedly **increases the risk** of the following disorders during adulthood: **posttraumatic stress disorder, depression, self-destructive and/or suicidal behavior, and substance abuse.** Almost all those with **dissociative identity disorder** (multiple personality disorder) have a history of sexual abuse as a child (classic board question).

Child Psychiatry

History

A 4-year-old boy is brought to see you by his mother at the request of the child's nursery school teacher. The mother reports that the child's behavior and mannerisms have always been concerning to her. She says he was born 7 weeks prematurely and did not say his first word until the age of 18 months. He seems socially withdrawn to her, often not responding to his name and rarely seeking her out. The mother also reports that her son likes to do the same things over and over again.

Since starting preschool, the boy's behavior has become more of an issue. He does not join in group activities, does not share toys, has difficulty communicating and interacting with other children, and occasionally displays hyperactive and repetitive behavior. Attempts at discipline or redirection when the child is acting inappropriately or engaging in repetitive behaviors are often met with hostility and, sometimes, combativeness. When he recently hit another child for no apparent reason, the teacher asked the mother to seek psychiatric consultation.

Interview/Exam

The patient avoids eye contact and has a very limited range of facial expression. His language skills are well below average for his age and characterized by unusual grammar and word usage. He frequently does not respond when asked direct questions. When given a chance to play with a toy, he repeatedly bangs it against the floor for several minutes until it is taken away from him and placed back on a shelf. Further attempts at questioning are futile, as the child is preoccupied with the toy, staring at it on the shelf and continuing to pretend to bang it on the floor.

Tests

None

Pathophysiology

Autism is now thought to be a result of both **genetic and environmental insults** as opposed to being a functional disorder. There is an **increased risk** of autism in **siblings,** and a high concordance rate among identical twins. In addition, autism is associated with an increased risk of other **congenital anomalies** and **perinatal complications, congenital rubella, phenylketonuria, fragile X syndrome, and tuberous sclerosis.** **Seizures** are common in autism, as are **EEG abnormalities** and, more recently, anatomic and functional brain abnormalities on radiologic imaging. **Males are affected more often** than females by a 4:1 ratio, but females tend to be more severely affected. The prevalence is roughly 1 in 3000. Autism tends to be a **lifelong** disorder, with two-thirds of affected adults still dependent on relatives or living in an institution.

Diagnosis & Treatment

Symptoms begin **before the age of 3.** The hallmarks of the disorder are: (1) **abnormalities in social interaction,** (2) **abnormalities of communication,** and (3) **restricted, repetitive, and stereotyped behavior and interests.** All three must be present to make the diagnosis.

Social abnormalities include failure to use eye contact, facial expression, posture, and gestures when interacting with others; **failure to develop friends;** inability or unwillingness to share; and a **lack of social and/or emotional reciprocity** during interactions. *Communication abnormalities* include a **delay or lack of spoken language,** failure to maintain conversation, and **unusual use of words or phrases,** including stereotyped or repetitive use of language. *Behavior abnormalities* include intense and/or abnormally focused interests, **compulsive adherence to rituals or routines,** and **repetitive and stereotyped body movements.** The **IQ is generally low,** with 40% of those affected having an IQ **below 50,** though 20% may have a normal nonverbal IQ.

Treatment is difficult, but includes psychotherapy for both child and family, and possibly adjunctive medications. **Antipsychotics** and **antidepressants** may help with aggressive behavior and compulsive symptoms, respectively.

More High-Yield Facts

The **idiot or autistic savant** is well portrayed in the movie "Rain Man" (consider seeing it if you have trouble understanding what makes a person autistic). These patients have a **specific gift** of memory, calculation, reading, or musical talent that is beyond the capability of a normal peer.

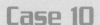

Case 10

Child Psychiatry

History

A mother is worried about her 6-year-old son because he "talks funny." She wants to know what treatments are available for the child's speech impediment, as it has started to affect his interactions with other children at school and has caused him a great deal of anxiety and embarrassment. She says the problem first began several months ago, but has gradually gotten worse. The boy is otherwise happy and healthy, and has no significant past medical or psychiatric history. He takes no medications.

Interview/Exam

The patient's speech is characterized by multiple sound and syllable repetitions (e.g., "I-I-I-I don't know"), and he frequently seems to make a substitution when he gets "stuck" on a problematic word or phrase. He is clearly frustrated with his speech difficulty and begins to cry. After calming him down, you find that he is an intelligent boy who is alert and appropriate. His vocabulary, word use, and syntax are normal for age. No other speech abnormalities are noted. The child is of normal height and weight for his age group, and he appears healthy.

Tests

None

Pathophysiology

Stuttering is thought to be due to a combination of genetic and environmental factors. A higher incidence is **seen in the family members** of affected persons. **Males are more commonly affected** than females by a 3:1 ratio. About **1% of the population** stutters at some point in their lives. Stuttering **often remits spontaneously before adulthood.**

Diagnosis & Treatment

Stuttering is characterized by **repetition of syllables and/or sounds,** including repetition of monosyllabic whole words (e.g., "I"), **sound prolongations, broken words, speech pauses,** and **word substitutions** to avoid problematic words. **Peak incidence** occurs in those **aged 2–7,** though symptoms may begin at other ages. Affected children often experience **anxiety, frustration, fear, embarrassment, and/or depression** related to their stuttering and may **avoid settings** that require them to speak. Stuttering is *not* considered a disorder unless **significant impairment** (e.g., academic or occupational difficulty, severe problems with communication) occurs. People who stutter may be teased or ridiculed by peers.

The important thing to remember is that **50–80%** of children who stutter will **recover spontaneously,** generally before adulthood. **Behavioral and speech therapy** are the currently favored treatments to help people learn to speak more effectively. In addition, adjunctive therapy to help people reduce anxiety and fear of stuttering may also aid in improving speech. Medications are generally *not* indicated, except to treat coexisting conditions (e.g., depression).

More High-Yield Facts

Stuttering is *not* thought to be caused by underlying anxiety; however, **stressful situations may exacerbate stuttering.**

Reassurance is often the best treatment in mild cases.

When the diagnosis is stuttering, the following generally are *not* present: problems with vocabulary, syntax, or grammar; breathing difficulties; a receptive or expressive aphasia. These findings may indicate another type of communication disorder.

Child Psychiatry

History

A 5-year-old boy is troubled by severe nightmares. The mother states that both she and her husband are awakened at least four times a week by a horrible scream, generally 2–3 hours after their son has fallen asleep. When they run to comfort him, he looks terrified and is generally screaming, sweating, and breathing rapidly. He is always confused, not knowing where he is or what is happening, for several minutes after his parents begin comforting him. The child never remembers what his nightmare was about and often goes right back to sleep, only to forget the entire episode the next morning. He has no past medical or psychiatric history and takes no regular medications.

Interview/Exam

Physical exam reveals no neurologic deficits or other abnormalities, and the patient is of normal height and weight for his age. He is alert and active, and seems to have normal cognitive development and intelligence for his age. The child says he thinks he might have bad dreams, but he doesn't remember them, and he seems happy and well adjusted; there are no signs of depression or irritability.

Tests

MRI of the brain: normal
EEG: normal

Pathophysiology

Sleep terror disorder affects **2–3%** of children, tends to **run in families,** and is **more common in boys** than girls. The disorder appears to have some relation to sleepwalking, and often the two coexist in affected patients. Polysomnography studies have shown that night terrors occur during **deep (stage 3 and 4) non-REM sleep,** distinguishing them from nightmares. Night terrors may reflect a minor neurological abnormality (though this has not been proven), given the association of symptoms with temporal lobe epilepsy.

Diagnosis & Treatment

Symptoms generally begin in children **aged 3–6 years.** Patients have episodes of **sudden awakening from sleep beginning with a panicky scream.** The awakenings generally occur during the **first one-third of the night** and usually last **< 10 minutes.** During this period of awakening, patients have **intense anxiety** accompanied by **autonomic signs** such as **tachycardia, rapid breathing, and sweating.** In addition, patients are **generally disoriented, confused, and/or unresponsive to attempts by others to comfort them.** Patients do *not* remember having a dream, though they may occasionally remember a single frightening image.

The episode terminates with the patient **falling back to sleep** or develops into a sleepwalking episode. **Patients have amnesia for the entire event.**

When symptoms first occur in adolescence or young adulthood (uncommon), they often reflect the development of **temporal lobe epilepsy.** It is therefore important to exclude this disorder as a cause of night terror symptoms. The **EEG is often abnormal** in temporal lobe epilepsy, while it is *normal in sleep terror disorder.*

Treatment is generally **supportive,** as the disorder tends to **resolve on its own by adolescence** if the onset is during childhood. Those with an onset during adolescence or young adulthood often have a **more chronic course. Psychotherapy** to explore possible stressors, family dynamics, and coping mechanisms may be useful. **Diazepam** is not routinely used, but can be given in severe cases; it often improves symptoms and may completely eliminate the attacks.

More High-Yield Facts

External stressors can **exacerbate or precipitate** the disorder, and **substance abuse** may cause the disorder in rare cases.

Psychiatry

History

A 27-year-old man comes to see you at the request of his new boss. The patient is not sure why he needs to see you, but his boss of 2 months says he is "a little off" and wants to make sure he is fit to handle his responsibilities at work. The patient works in a mailroom sorting mail. He has no medical or psychiatric history and takes no medications. The patient denies drug or alcohol use. His father was diagnosed as schizophrenic.

Interview/Exam

The patient is difficult to communicate with because of his peculiar way of thinking and speaking—vague, circumstantial, and overly elaborate. He has a somewhat constricted affect and seems unconcerned when he admits that he has no close friends other than his mother. He states that people "are all the same, all made of wood." The patient has a strong belief in the occult and mentions several superstitions that have guided his behavior (e.g., never wears black clothes on a Monday) since he was an adolescent. His mannerisms are eccentric, but consistent and fairly organized.

The patient denies hallucinations and does not seem to harbor any obvious delusions. He denies depression and suicidal ideation. The patient's mother calls to speak with you and says that her son's behavior has not changed recently; he has always been somewhat eccentric, but "never caused any trouble."

Tests

None

Pathophysiology

The etiology of this disorder is at least partially **genetic,** as there is an increased twin concordance and increased incidence of SPD and of **schizophrenia** in first-degree relatives. Some with SPD may in fact become schizophrenic later in life. Like all personality disorders, the pattern of maladaptive traits is **lifelong,** often beginning in adolescence.

Diagnosis & Treatment

Those with SPD have a lifelong pattern of a **reduced capacity for close relationships and odd thoughts, perception, communication, and behavior.** Diagnostic criteria include: ideas (not delusions) of reference, **bodily illusions,** suspiciousness, **inappropriate and/or constricted affect,** social anxiety due to paranoid fears, and a **lack of close friends** (other than first-degree relatives). In addition, **odd thinking and speech** are classic (e.g., **vague, circumstantial, stereotypical, overly elaborate, or metaphorical speech**). **Odd beliefs that influence behavior,** such as **superstitions, the occult,** and personal powers of **clairvoyance or telepathy,** are also classic and are likely to be mentioned in a Step 2 question.

Note that these patients are **not psychotic** like schizophrenic patients (e.g., no hallucinations or true delusions; behavior and thought eccentric/odd, but not grossly disorganized). Brief psychosis may occur under severe stress, but the episode is short lived. **Up to 10%** of affected patients eventually **commit suicide.**

Treatment includes **psychotherapy** and **antipsychotics** if needed for ideas of reference, illusions, or paranoia. As with all personality disorders, treatment often is not very effective.

More High-Yield Facts

It can be tough to keep straight all of the psychiatric diagnoses with the "schiz-" prefix, which (of course) makes for great board questions.
• Patients with SPD are similar to patients with *schizophrenia* in that they have odd beliefs, thoughts, speech, and behavior, *but* only schizophrenic patients are truly **psychotic.**
• *Schizoid personality disorder* patients are classic "loners" who do not want relationships, but have **relatively normal** beliefs, thoughts, speech, and behavior.
• *Schizoaffective* patients essentially have **schizophrenia** coexisting with a **mood disorder.**

Psychiatry

History

A 37-year-old woman is concerned because she "feels lousy" all the time. She almost always feels tired and overworked and often has trouble concentrating. She says that her symptoms began about 10 years ago, but she has never sought psychiatric help. The patient reports feeling depressed just about every day, and hardly ever feels as though things are going well in her life. She denies suicidal ideation, weight loss, or any discrete episodes of particularly severe symptoms. She is an accountant and has been with the same company for 12 years; she believes she has been able to perform her work duties adequately. Family history is significant for depression in her father and one of her paternal uncles.

Interview/Exam

The patient is alert, oriented, and intelligent. Her mood is depressed, but she is not tearful. She is pessimistic and seems to have a fairly low self-esteem. Her cognitive and reasoning abilities are intact, and she denies hallucinations or delusions. Her thoughts and speech are organized and logical. Her weight is normal for height.

Tests

Hemoglobin: 14 g/dL (normal 12–16)
Thyroid-stimulating hormone: 2.3 μU/mL (normal 0.5–5)
Erythrocyte sedimentation rate: 8 mm/hr (normal 1–20)
Calcium: 9.2 mg/dL (normal 8.5–10.5)

Pathophysiology

Dysthymic disorder is thought to be caused by a combination of **genetics and environment.** Many patients have a **family history of mood disorders.** The disorder is thought to affect **up to 5% of the population** and is **more common in females,** younger adults, those who are single, and those with low incomes.

Diagnosis & Treatment

The hallmark of this disorder is the **nearly constant presence of a depressed mood** without full-blown major depression. **At least 2 years of steady symptoms** (depressed mood more days than not) must be present to make this diagnosis in adults. Additional symptoms include **appetite changes, sleep disturbances, low energy, fatigue, low self-esteem, poor concentration, difficulty making decisions, and feelings of hopelessness.** These symptoms are all less dramatic and more constant than in major depression. By definition, these patients *cannot* have a history of hypomania or mania episodes (which would make them cyclothymic or bipolar, respectively).

Long-term **substance abuse** can cause symptoms nearly identical to dysthymic disorder, and many patients with dysthymic disorder abuse substances as a form of "self-medication." In general, *don't* diagnose dysthymic disorder if substance abuse has coexisted for the entire time symptoms have been present. (Instead, this would be called a mood disorder secondary to substance abuse.)

The best treatment is a combination of **psychotherapy and antidepressant medications** (usually serotonin-specific reuptake inhibitors or bupropion). Treatment is difficult given the long-standing nature of most people's symptoms.

More High-Yield Facts

Mood Disorders 101

Dysthymia: chronic, mild depression
Cyclothymia: mild depression alternating with hypomania
Biploar I: mania +/− depression
Bipolar II: hypomania alternating with major depression
"Double depression": major depression superimposed on coexisting dysthymia

Psychiatry

History

A 39-year-old man comes to the emergency department complaining of severe low back pain and requesting meperidine for pain. He says he twisted his back while climbing up a ladder and has been in excruciating pain for the last week. He says he saw a doctor at a clinic for this problem, and was given a prescription for meperidine, but he lost it. The patient states that no other pain relievers are effective at reducing the pain. He denies any significant past medical or psychiatric history and takes no regular medications. The patient denies drug or alcohol use, but he smokes about one pack of cigarettes per day.

Interview/Exam

The patient is sweating and irritable, and yawns several times during the interview and exam. His pupils are dilated, but symmetric and reactive. You note multiple scabs on his forearms, suspicious for needle marks. During your exam, the patient seems to have a heightened sensitivity to pain, complaining of pain whenever you perform any type of palpation. He winces when you touch his lower back, but when you distract him, the same palpation does not elicit any complaints. Straight leg raise is negative, and no muscle spasm is present. Neurologic exam is normal. The patient's irritability increases; he becomes restless and repeatedly asks for pain relief.

Tests

X-ray of the lumbosacral spine: normal

Pathophysiology

Roughly 1% of the U.S. population has tried heroin, the most widely abused opioid. About 500,000 people are dependent on opioids, and half of these individuals live in **New York City.** Opioid dependence is **more common in males** than females by a 3:1 ratio, and most addicts are **ages 30–45.** Heroin is generally either injected (intravenously or subcutaneously) or snorted (though prescription opiates are often taken orally). Those who inject have a high risk of **hepatitis B/C/D** and **HIV,** as well as other complications such as **endocarditis** (classically right-sided valves affected), skin infections/abscesses, and **criminal activity** including theft and prostitution to pay for their drug habit.

Diagnosis & Treatment

Heroin intoxication causes **euphoria, altered mood, drowsiness, psychomotor retardation, perceptual disturbances, decreased sensation of pain, and impaired memory and attention.** Many report being in a **dream-like state.** Other signs include **pupillary constriction** (miosis) and **slurred speech. Coma** can occur with overdose.

Withdrawal results in **pupillary dilatation** (mydriasis), **fever/sweating, gooseflesh** (piloerection), **dysphoria, nausea/vomiting/diarrhea, lacrimation, rhinorrhea, muscle aches, yawning, insomnia, irritability, restlessness, and heightened pain sensitivity.** Those withdrawing from opioids feel miserable and often act as though they are going to die, but opioid **withdrawal is almost never life-threatening.**

Treatment is complex, as with most addictions, and **relapses are common.** Opioid antagonists, primarily **naltrexone** but also **mixed agonist-antagonist agents** such as buprenorphine, can be given orally long-term to prevent intoxicating effects when opioids are used. **Naloxone** can be given intravenously in the event of an **opioid overdose. Methadone is controversial,** but the theory behind it is to substitute a long-acting lower dose of a prescription opioid agonist to allow a person to return to productivity while gradually decreasing the dose over time. Shorter-acting opioids cause withdrawal symptoms that are more intense and begin sooner after the last dose.

More High-Yield Facts

About 15% of people with opioid dependence attempt to **commit suicide** at least once.

Giving an opioid addict **an opioid antagonist can precipitate immediate withdrawal symptoms.**

Psychiatry

History

A 28-year-old man is brought into the emergency department by his mother for high fevers, sweating, and confusion. She also says he has stopped talking. The mother says the symptoms began early this morning and quickly got worse. Her son lives with her and was diagnosed with schizophrenia 2 weeks ago. She states that he has not been exposed to any sick people lately; his only medication is haloperidol; and he has no other medical problems. According to the mother, her son has never used illicit drugs or alcohol.

Interview/Exam

T: 106°F   BP: 172/98   P: 106/min   RR: 18/min

The patient is diaphoretic and mute, apparently unable to answer questions, and appears frightened. His level of consciousness is decreased, and his ability to pay attention to you is limited; he is unable to follow commands. No photophobia is detected, and the patient's pupils are equal and reactive. Forced neck flexion does not seem to cause any discomfort. His chest is clear to auscultation, and no cardiac murmurs are appreciated. His abdomen is soft and nontender. Musculoskeletal exam reveals muscular rigidity, and the patient does not move his extremities when asked, though he withdraws slightly from painful stimuli.

Tests

Hemoglobin: 16 g/dL (normal 14–18)
White blood cells: 15,800/μL (normal 4500–11,000)
Sodium: 140 meq/L (normal 135–145)
Potassium: 4.9 meq/L (normal 3.5–5.0)
Creatine phosphokinase (CPK): 5200 u/L (normal 17–48)
CK-MB fraction: less than 3%
Creatinine: 1.1 mg/dL (normal 0.6–1.5)
Urinalysis: negative for bacteria, glucose, and white and red blood cells; 1+ proteinuria; positive myoglobinuria
Lumbar puncture, cerebrospinal fluid analysis: no organisms detected, normal cell count, normal glucose and protein levels, normal opening pressure
EKG: sinus tachycardia
Thyroid stimulating hormone: 2.3 μU/mL (normal 0.5–5)
CT scan of the head: negative

Pathophysiology

NMS is thought to occur in roughly 1% of those who are prescribed classic anti-psychotics. The mechanism is not well understood, but NMS can also occur in those with Parkinson's disease if their dopamine agonist medication is abruptly discontinued. NMS classically occurs **shortly after** a person is started on an antipsychotic, but can also arise **after years of use.** NMS is thought to be much **less common with newer-generation antipsychotic agents** (e.g., risperidone, olanzapine).

Diagnosis & Treatment

The classic pentad of NMS is **high fever (up to 107°F), high CPK (often > 1000 u/L), muscular rigidity, altered mental status,** and **a history of antipsychotic medication use. Diaphoresis,** dysphagia, tremor, incontinence, mutism (i.e., inability to talk), **tachycardia, elevated and/or labile blood pressure,** and **leukocytosis** are also common. **Myoglobinuria** may be noted on urinalysis, and liver function test results may be elevated. Other etiologies must be excluded, such as encephalitis, but the boards will present you with a classic case.

Treatment begins with **stopping the antipsychotic.** Supportive measures, such as **cooling blankets, IV fluids, and electrolyte correction** are the mainstays of therapy in most cases. **Dantrolene** (also used in malignant hyperthermia, which is somewhat similar) and **dopamine agonists** (usually **bromocriptine)** can be used in severe cases to reduce mortality. Mortality even with intensive treatment is estimated to be about **15%.**

More High-Yield Facts

Other Antipsychotic Side-Effects*

- Parkinsonism: classic symptoms such as resting tremor and rigidity. Most common in **elderly females.** Treat with **anticholinergics** (e.g., diphenhydramine, benztropine, trihexyphenidyl).
- Acute dystonia: **muscle spasms** (e.g., may see torticollis, jaw muscle spasm/ trismus, or impaired swallowing/speaking), **tongue protrusion,** and/or **sustained eye deviation** (oculogyric crisis). Most common in **younger men after the 1st dose.** Treat with **anticholinergics.**
- Akathisia: **restlessness** characterized by **pacing, fidgeting, and/or inability to sit or stand still** for more than a few minutes. Treat by reducing the dose or switching to a newer agent and/or a **beta-blocker.**
- Tardive dyskinesia: happens **after many years** of treatment. **Choreiform movements, athetoid movements,** and/or **rhythmic, stereotyped movements** may occur. **Abnormal oral, tongue,** and/or **facial movements** are classic. Treat by switching to newer-generation agent.

*Less common with newer-generation, atypical agents

Psychiatry

History

A 19-year-old woman seeks a referral to a plastic surgeon. She would like to have rhinoplasty because her nose is "way too big." The patient mentions that she is having trouble attracting male attention because of her nose and notices people staring at her nose in public places. She has been staying at home more and more frequently due to her feelings about her nose. She has tried various creams and make-up to make her nose appear smaller, without success.

The patient has no significant medical or psychiatric history, though she does admit to fairly frequent symptoms of depression. She denies suicidal ideation, does not use illicit drugs, and only rarely drinks alcohol.

Interview/Exam

The patient is alert, oriented, and intelligent. Her attention and concentration seem normal. Her thoughts are well organized and she denies hallucination or delusions. Her nose is well proportioned in relation to her face, and is actually on the small side! You notice that the patient frequently tries to cover her nose with her hand when she looks at you. At one point during the interview, she asks you if you are staring at her nose. No other abnormalities are detected.

Tests

None

Pathophysiology

BDD is a **preoccupation with an imagined defect** in physical appearance or an **exaggerated, distorted perception of a minor flaw** or defect in physical appearance. It typically begins in those **aged 15–20** and is **more common in females** than males. Affected people are usually **unmarried.** BDD is fairly common, and one study estimated that at least 2% of patients presenting to a plastic surgery clinic had this disorder. A **family history of mood disorders** is usual, suggesting a possible genetic link.

Diagnosis & Treatment

People with this disorder have a normal appearance or only a minor defect or flaw, but **believe they have a severe physical deformity.** Classically, they **seek medical or surgical treatment** for the imagined/exaggerated defect. The usual location of an imagined defect is the **hair, nose, or skin.** The eyes, head, and face are other common locations, though any body part may be involved, or overall body shape may be the primary concern. Many patients "switch" from one imagined defect to another. BDD causes clinically **significant distress or functional impairment** (e.g., constant worrying or paranoia about the defect, staying home to avoid personal contact).

Patients often have **ideas of reference** (e.g., think people are always noticing or staring at the imagined physical flaw), constantly check the mirror to examine the flaw, and **attempt to hide** it (e.g., cover it with clothes or makeup).

Avoid medical or surgical treatment, as it almost always fails to eradicate BDD. **Antidepressant medications** (usually serotonin-specific reuptake inhibitors) are effective in many cases, along with adjunctive psychotherapy. **Coexisting depression, anxiety, and/or psychosis are common** and may also require treatment.

More High-Yield Facts

Up to 20% of affected patients may eventually **attempt suicide** and this is thought to be partially related to the very high incidence ($\sim$ 90% of patients) of coexisting depression.

Symptoms are usually **chronic** and may wax and wane if the condition is left untreated.

Psychiatry

History

A 31-year-old woman has been rushed to the emergency department via ambulance after trying to commit suicide by cutting her wrists with a razor. She says she wanted to harm herself after having a fight with her live-in girlfriend. The patient says her girlfriend, who she has been dating on and off for 6 months, is an "evil monster." The woman relates chronic feelings of emptiness and boredom and admits to intermittent drug and alcohol abuse to "numb" her feelings. Social history includes multiple past sexual partners, both male and female, without any sustained relationships. Occupational history includes numerous unrelated, menial jobs, none of which was held for more than a few months. Family history is significant for substance abuse and depression in the patient's mother. Chart review reveals multiple suicide gestures over the past 5 years.

Interview/Exam

The patient is alert, oriented, and somewhat hostile at first. Her affect is labile, and during the interview she vacillates between anger and tears, with episodes of laughter in between. She says she previously had a therapist who was "an angel, the most perfect man in the world," but she stopped seeing him for financial reasons. The patient relates a fairly chaotic history of interpersonal relationships dating back to adolescence. Examination of her wrists reveals multiple, shallow, superficial cuts consistent with the action of a razorblade. The patient tells you that she had to cut her wrists to keep her girlfriend from leaving her.

Tests

None

Borderline personality disorder

Pathophysiology

Borderline personality disorder is estimated to affect roughly 1% of the population and is **twice as common in females.** Depression and substance abuse are common in first-degree relatives. As with all personality disorders, the traits of the disorder are generally lifelong in nature, often starting in adolescence. Other terms for borderline personality disorder—**ambulatory schizophrenia and emotionally unstable personality disorder**—help define it.

Diagnosis & Treatment

The hallmarks of borderline personality disorder are **impulsivity** and **instability of relationships, self-image, and affect.** Patients will go to great lengths to avoid real or imagined **threats of abandonment** and often have a history of **recurrent suicidal behavior/gestures/threats or self-mutilating behavior.** Chronic feelings of **boredom and/or emptiness** are classic. Patients also usually engage in **splitting,** which is when a person or thing is either "all good" (overly valued and respected) or "all bad" (overly loathed and devalued). The patient often **shifts allegiances** (e.g., a person goes from being viewed as an "angel" to a "devil"), sometimes in the course of a few minutes.

"Micropsychotic" episodes describe fleeting symptoms of psychosis that may last only a few minutes and are often brought out by stress. The affect is generally **labile,** with patients alternating between **intense anger/temper tantrums** and crying or laughter. Impulsivity may take the form of **promiscuous sex, out-of-control spending, substance abuse, or binge eating.** Patients also have a **markedly unstable and shifting sense of self,** which may be manifest by **bisexuality** and/or occupational or educational uncertainty. In all, patient **behavior is highly unpredictable.**

Treatment is difficult, but includes **psychotherapy** plus **adjunctive medications** (e.g., antidepressants, mood stabilizers, antipsychotics) if needed for specific for coexisting or dominant symptoms.

More High-Yield Facts

Recurrent self-mutilation and/or suicidal gestures or attempts is classic for borderline personality disorder, as are splitting, feelings of chronic emptiness, and chaotic relationships.

These patients *do not* have formal psychosis or thought disorders (distinguishes from schizophrenia) and generally have **normal intelligence.**

Psychiatry

History

A 27-year-old woman complains of frequent tension headaches, which she thinks are related to stress. She says her stress is mostly self-imposed, as she is constantly worrying about her job, home, finances, boyfriend, and pets. She claims her headaches and other symptoms began roughly 3 years ago and occur nearly every day. The patient also mentions frequently feeling "on edge," irritable, and restless. This causes her to have difficulty concentrating and leaves her feeling fatigued most of the time. The patient works as a secretary in a law firm and feels her work is affected by her symptoms, though she has never been reprimanded for her performance. She denies drug or alcohol abuse.

Interview/Exam

The patient is alert, oriented, and intelligent. She seems restless and anxious and mentions difficulty sleeping. Her memory and concentration objectively seem intact. During the physical exam, the patient describe multiple somatic problems, such as frequent shortness of breath, dry throat, occasional palpitations, and diarrhea. The eyes and oropharynx appear normal, and no thyroid abnormalities are palpable. Cardiac and lung exams are unremarkable. No abdominal tenderness is present, and bowel sounds are normal. No neurologic or skin abnormalities are identified. Your nurse enters the room toward the end of the exam and the patient is visibly startled, gasping and clutching her chest until she realizes who the person is.

Tests

Thyroid-stimulating hormone: 2.6 μU/mL (normal 0.5–5)
Calcium: 9 mg/dL (normal 8.5–10.5)
Hemoglobin: 13 mg/dL (normal 12–16)
Urine toxicology screen: negative for illicit drugs
Glucose: 86 mg/dL (normal fasting 70–110)
EKG: normal sinus rhythm with no abnormalities

Pathophysiology

Generalized anxiety disorder is fairly common, with an estimated prevalence of roughly **5%.** It is **twice as common in females,** and patients usually come to the attention of a clinician in their **20s.** A combination of biologic and psychological factors is thought to be causative. At least **half** of affected patients have another coexisting mental disorder, usually a **phobia, panic disorder, or depressive disorder.**

Diagnosis & Treatment

People with generalized anxiety disorder are **constantly worrying and/or anxious.** This worry extends to **multiple aspects** of the patient's life, including relationships, finances, and career. Patients classically describe **feeling restless, "keyed up," or "on edge."** They also often complain of **fatigue, difficulty concentrating, irritability, muscle tension** (tension headaches are classic), and **difficulty sleeping. Somatic complaints, such as palpitations, dry throat, shortness of breath, excessive sweating, and diarrhea, are common.** Due to constant anxiety and worry, patients are "on the lookout" for trouble (hypervigilance or hyperalertness) and classically are **startled very easily.**

Symptoms must be present for **at least 6 months** to make the diagnosis, but most patients report several years of symptoms by the time they seek medical attention. Patients often initially present to non-psychiatric clinicians for somatic complaints. **Hyperthyroidism and stimulant or caffeine abuse must be ruled out,** as they can cause identical symptoms.

Treatment includes **psychotherapy plus medications. Benzodiazepines** are effective but **sedating,** and **tolerance** and **dependence** can develop. Therefore, **avoid long-term** treatment with benzodiazepines. **Buspirone** and **serotonin-specific reuptake inhibitors** (SSRIs) are also effective and do not cause the same side-effect problems as benzodiazepines, but **both require a few weeks to begin working.** Some clinicians start treatment with a benzodiazepine plus an SSRI or buspirone, then **taper** the benzodiazepine in a few weeks once the other agent has had a chance to start working.

More High-Yield Facts

Patients with generalized anxiety disorder worry about everything all the time and *do not* have discrete, dramatic episodes/attacks as those with panic disorder do. **Anxiety and depression** can be difficult to distinguish, and they **often coexist** in the same patient.

Psychiatry

History

A 26-year-old man is brought to the emergency department by his friend, who says he's been "acting crazy." The friend reports that the patient was smoking marijuana a few hours ago, and he thinks it may have been "laced" with something, as the patient started acting bizarrely several minutes later. The friend does not think the patient has any medical problems or takes any medications. He states that he has known the patient for 15 years and he has never acted this way before.

Interview/Exam

T: 100.1°F   BP: 160/92   P: 98/min   RR: 16/min

The patient is agitated and paranoid and refuses to answer questions. You noted that he was somewhat ataxic as he walked into the exam room. He occasionally speaks out, generally slurring his words and making little sense. At one point the patient begins swinging violently at some imaginary object. He calms down a few minutes later and is able to cooperate somewhat with the rest of the exam.

Eye exam reveals horizontal and vertical nystagmus. His skin is flushed and warm. Chest and cardiac exams are normal, and no abdominal abnormalities are appreciated. His reflexes are brisk and symmetric. Mental status exam reveals difficulty concentrating, poor judgment, and disordered thought process. The patient frequently seems confused and intermittently becomes agitated and paranoid.

Tests

Urine drug screen: pending

Pathophysiology

PCP ("angel dust") was originally developed as a **dissociative anesthetic** and is still used in some parts of the world for veterinary procedures. It works partly via **antagonism of N-methyl-D-aspartate (NMDA) receptors and activation of dopamine receptors.** PCP abuse is most commonly seen in **males aged 20–40** who also abuse other substances. PCP is usually smoked or ingested orally. The drugs' effect has been used as a **model for schizophrenia,** and the clinical state of intoxication can strongly resemble the symptoms and signs of psychosis.

Diagnosis & Treatment

PCP intoxication can cause **belligerence, aggressive/violent and unpredictable behavior, impulsiveness, agitation, and impaired judgment and functioning.** Visual or auditory **hallucinations** may occur, and the affect may be **labile.**

Physical signs of PCP use include **vertical and/or horizontal nystagmus** (classic), **hyperthermia, hypertension, increased heart rate, muscular rigidity, decreased pain sensation, ataxia, slurred speech/dysarthria,** and/or **hyperacusis.** Overdose can cause **convulsions, coma, or death.** Physical dependence does *not* occur, and withdrawal is *not* dangerous.

Treatment is generally **supportive.** "Talking patients down" occasionally helps, and placing them in a **stimulus-free environment** (e.g., a quiet, dark room) can help reduce agitation. **Benzodiazepines** and **antipsychotics** are often needed acutely to help control patients' behavior. In severe overdose, **acidification of the urine** with ammonium chloride may help speed elimination. Careful monitoring of vital signs and renal function is needed with an overdose, as severe **hypertension, respiratory arrest, convulsions, and rhabdomyolysis** may occur and require urgent treatment. Drug-induced psychosis may last **several days or even weeks.**

More High-Yield Facts

PCP's effects are somewhat similar to LSD, but individuals taking PCP are often **more violent and agitated,** and many of the physical signs (e.g., nystagmus, muscular rigidity) of PCP use do *not* occur with LSD intoxication.

Ketamine ("special K") is another dissociative anesthetic still used in some clinical situations that has become a drug of abuse, though symptoms tend to be milder, and violence and agitation are rare. Its half-life is also much shorter (2 hours, versus 20 hours for PCP).

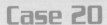

Psychiatry

History

A 29-year-old woman is brought to the emergency department by the police after they found her running naked across a busy street carrying a large wooden cross. The patient was agitated and had to be handcuffed. She kept referring to her "mission for the Lord" and demanded to be set free multiple times. The patient keeps insisting that her name is "the agent."

The patient's husband arrives after being notified by a neighbor that the police had picked up his wife. He says she has never acted this way before and that her symptoms came on gradually over the past 2 weeks. The changes began with the patient becoming unusually energetic and having a decreased need for sleep. She started to talk more and more, though she is usually a fairly quiet and introspective person. A few days ago, she suddenly became preoccupied with religious ideas, though she has not practiced her religion in years. Apparently, the patient left the house last night while her husband was sleeping, not telling him where she was going. The man claims that his wife has no medical problems, takes no medications, and does not use alcohol or illicit drugs.

Interview/Exam

The patient is extremely talkative, and her speech is disorganized and rapid. She claims to be an "agent of God" who has been sent to deliver a coded message to the leaders of the world. She says that she speaks with God almost constantly and that she hasn't slept in several days, as she has "too much to do." The patient is easily distracted, frequently interrupts your questions, and jumps from one topic to another without pausing when speaking.

Tests

Urine drug screen: negative
Ethanol level: undetectable
Thyroid-stimulating hormone: 2 μU/mL (normal 0.5–5)
Calcium: 9.1 mg/dL (normal 8.5–10.5)
Sodium: 140 meq/L (normal 135–145)
Creatinine: 0.9 mg/dL (normal 0.6–1.5)

Pathophysiology

Bipolar disorder is estimated to affect **1%** of the population and has an equal incidence in males and females. The average **age of onset** is **21–30** years. Most individuals come to medical attention because of severe impairment caused by a manic episode, which is all that is needed to make the diagnosis (though alternating manic and depressed episodes are classic). There is a strong **genetic component,** and first-degree relatives of those affected are **10 times more likely to have a mood disorder.** When one parent is bipolar, a child has a 25% chance of developing a mood disorder; if both parents are affected, the chance is 50–75%.

Diagnosis & Treatment

Mania is characterized by a **persistently elevated, expansive, and/or irritable mood.** Patients may have **inflated self-esteem** or be **grandiose,** and classically have a **decreased need for sleep.** They are often **talkative,** and speech is classically **pressured** (you may have to wait forever for a turn to speak). **Flight of ideas** (rapid topic shifting with each topic only loosely connected to the previous one) and being **easily distracted** are also common. Patients typically indulge in pleasurable activities **without regard for consequences,** such as **promiscuous sex, shopping sprees,** and **foolish business investments.**

Bipolar disorder may comprise only manic episodes, or mania alternating with depressive episodes. **Depression is not required** for a diagnosis of bipolar I disorder. **Psychotic symptoms** may dominate the clinical picture in patients with more severe manic episodes. **Schizoaffective disorder** can be tough to distinguish, but is characterized by psychotic symptoms **without mood symptoms** at some point.

Treatment involves psychotherapy, **mood stabilizers** (e.g., lithium or valproic acid), and **antipsychotics** and/or **sedatives** (e.g., benzodiazepines) if needed. Olanzapine is also now FDA-approved as a treatment for acute mania. Hospitalization (involuntary if necessary) is often required for a manic episode, as patients may harm themselves or others. Other mood stabilizers, such as carbamazepine, lamotrigine, and gabapentin, are considered second-line agents by most clinicians.

More High-Yield Facts

Many now use **valproic acid** (watch for **liver toxicity)** instead of lithium, as lithium has more frequent adverse effects (**renal damage/diabetes insipidus, thyroid abnormalities, tremor**).

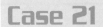

Psychiatry

History

A 32-year-old man is referred to your office by his parole officer for evaluation. The man was recently arrested for credit card fraud and has a long history of arrests beginning at the age of 10 for multiple crimes, including theft, assault, fraud, and arson. He has no significant past medical or psychiatric history and takes no regular medications. He admits to drinking alcohol on a daily basis and has blacked out and passed out secondary to alcohol use on innumerable occasions. The patient has also experimented with many illicit drugs and has sold them in the past. He says he has children with several different women, but doesn't keep in contact with any of them or pay child support. The patient's father was an alcoholic and left home when the patient was 3 years old.

Interview/Exam

The patient is alert, oriented, and intelligent. He is fairly pleasant to talk with and does not seem anxious or depressed. His thoughts are organized and rational. When asked about his arrests, the patient avoids the issue and pleasantly changes the subject multiple times. When confronted more directly and vigorously, the patient becomes defensive and hostile, refusing to answer your questions. He appears to lack remorse for his crimes and for his behavior regarding his children.

Tests

None

Antisocial personality disorder

Pathophysiology

Antisocial personality disorder affects roughly **2%** of the population and is **three times more common in males.** The classic description is a **con-man without a conscience.** In **prison populations,** the prevalence of this disorder may be as high as 75%. A **genetic basis** is believed to be at least partly responsible, as the disorder is five times more common in first-degree relatives of affected males.

Diagnosis & Treatment

Those with antisocial personality disorder have a **basic disregard for the rights of others** and often **violate others' rights without remorse. Acts of criminality** are almost universal, and **deceitfulness, lying, and conning others** are diagnostic criteria. Patients are often **impulsive, fail to plan ahead, have a reckless disregard for the safety of others and themselves, lack remorse, and are consistently irresponsible** (e.g., fail to honor financial, work, and parental obligations). **Spousal/child abuse, promiscuity, and drunk driving** are common, and patients are rarely employed for any significant length of time.

Affected individuals **cannot be trusted** to perform any task or obey any moral standard. Interestingly, they are **superficially charming,** especially when interacting with the opposite sex. However, if their demands are not met or they are confronted about their activities, they are quick to reveal **underlying rage and hostility.** Affected patients use their charm to **manipulate** others (e.g., get money or convince others to fulfill their needs). There is an increased incidence of **alcoholism (75%)/substance abuse, depression,** and **somatization** in these individuals. A family history of alcoholism is common.

Treatment is **rarely effective,** but psychotherapy and medications to treat specific symptoms (e.g., depression) may be of some use. Symptoms often lessen somewhat with age. Those affected are at **increased risk of suicide.**

More High-Yield Facts

A **conduct disorder,** which is the *pediatric equivalent* of antisocial disorder, **must technically be present** to make the diagnosis of antisocial personality disorder. Look for a history of running away, setting fires, cruelty to animals, lying, theft, fighting, substance abuse, and other illegal activities before the age of 15.

People with antisocial personality disorder **know right from wrong** (i.e., not criminally insane), but they don't care and seem to enjoy breaking rules.

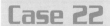

Psychiatry

History

A 32-year-old man comes to the emergency department complaining of blood in his urine this morning. There is no history of hematuria in the past. The patient does not have any other symptoms and does not take any medications. He denies using alcohol or illicit drugs, and his family history is unremarkable. He is employed as a phlebotomist.

Interview/Exam

Vital signs are normal. The physical examination is unremarkable, with no abdominal masses or tenderness noted. The nurse comes into the room at the end of the exam and grabs the patient's clothes to move them into a designated patient storage area. A bottle of pills falls out of the pants pockets. The bottle is half-full of warfarin tablets. The patient denies any knowledge of the pills, and claims that the nurse planted them there.

Out in the hall, the nurse mentions that she has seen the patient before at another hospital where she used to work and thinks he was admitted there for hematuria as well. A call to the other hospital confirms the admission for hematuria and a lab profile consistent with excessive warfarin use. The patient left the hospital against medical advice. When you return to the patient to confront him with this information, he is gone.

Tests

Urinalysis: positive for red blood cells, otherwise normal

Pathophysiology

Factitious disorder is said to occur when a person pretends to be ill in order to assume the sick role. It seems to be **most common among hospital and health-care workers** and is slightly more common in **males.** The etiology may be related to childhood abuse, **childhood hospitalization,** and/or rejecting parents. Symptoms often begin in **early adulthood.**

Diagnosis & Treatment

Patients may fake any type of physical or psychiatric illness, and their **medical background** helps them to be convincing. Using insulin to cause hypoglycemia or anticoagulants to cause bleeding are classic case scenarios. The boards will have to give you some indication that the illness is being faked.

The hallmark of this disorder is that the individual's only goal in faking illness is **to assume the role of a patient** (i.e., **the sick role**). There is **no financial or other secondary gain** (e.g., disability, time off from work, avoiding jail), which if present would change the diagnosis to malingering. However, symptoms are **produced voluntarily,** separating factitious disorder from **somatization disorder and hypochondriasis,** in which symptoms are *not* produced intentionally. Patients with **conversion disorder** are not medically sophisticated (their symptoms are not convincing), and there is usually an obvious **recent emotional conflict** that triggered the symptoms. In addition, only factitious disorder patients are generally **willing to submit to painful or potentially mutilating procedures.**

Patients often have a history of **repeated visits to different hospitals or clinicians in different areas,** to avoid detection. Some patients may undergo painful procedures and even major surgery. Those affected often have **normal intelligence** and lack a formal thought disorder.

Treatment is difficult and rarely successful. **Early recognition** of the disorder can help prevent potentially dangerous treatments from being given. Try to **avoid direct confrontation** or exposure of the patient's motivations, at least initially, because this approach often causes him or her to leave the hospital.

More High-Yield Facts

Both malingerers and persons with factitious disorder **intentionally produce symptoms,** but they are looking for **different rewards** (malingerers want to get money or avoid work, jail, or responsibility; persons with factitious disorder simply want to be a patient).

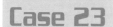

Case 23

Psychiatry

History

A mother has made an appointment for her 16-year-old daughter because she is worried about the girl's frequent crying spells. The mother says that ever since her daughter broke-up with her boyfriend 1 month ago, she has been acting sad and depressed. The mother says the child brought home her first "C" grade and hasn't been studying or talking to her friends as much as usual since the break-up. The patient is normally an "A" student and very outgoing. The patient has no significant past medical or psychiatric history, takes no medications, and denies any history of drug or alcohol use.

Interview/Exam

The girl appears healthy and well nourished, but her mood is tearful. She admits to feeling sad and depressed since the break-up with her boyfriend of 4 months. The patient mentions that her schoolwork has slipped. She has not lost any weight or had any significant sleep disturbance. She denies suicidal ideation and does not seem to have significant psychomotor retardation. She also denies hallucinations and delusions. Her memory and concentration are normal, and she seems to have above-average intelligence.

Tests

Urine pregnancy test: negative

Adjustment disorder with depressed mood

Pathophysiology

Adjustment disorder describes a reaction to (often) normal life stressors that is disproportionate to the stressor or severe enough to impair functioning. It is an extremely **common** disorder and is often seen in medically ill patients in the hospital. **Females are affected twice as often as males.** Those who are **unmarried** and **adolescents** have an **increased risk** of the disorder.

Diagnosis & Treatment

Patients have an **identifiable life stressor** that is *not* life threatening, such as a **divorce/relationship break-up, school problem, moving to a new environment, or financial problems.** They develop emotional and/or behavioral symptoms in response **within 3 months** of the event. The response to the stressor is either **in excess of what would normally be expected** or causes **impairment in social, occupational and/or academic functioning.** Symptoms usually last < 3 months.

The adjustment disorder diagnosis is often made with a specifier, such as **"with depressed mood," "with anxiety,"** or "unspecified." The normality of the stressor and the **absence of flashbacks** separates adjustment disorder from posttraumatic stress disorder (PTSD). Patients with anxiety or depression do *not* meet the full-blown criteria for an anxiety disorder or major depression. Do *not* diagnose adjustment disorder in a person experiencing grief (bereavement) from the loss of a loved one.

The treatment of choice for adjustment disorder is **psychotherapy. Medications** may be used briefly in severe cases to reduce depression or anxiety.

More High-Yield Facts

Patients with **PTSD** have been through **life-threatening trauma** outside the normal realm of human experience, such as rape, war, a car accident, or a natural disaster. Those with adjustment disorder have been through a **fairly normal life event.**

Occasionally, adjustment disorder can lead to **conduct disturbances,** such as vandalism or fighting, or other maladaptive responses, such as **denial of serious physical illness** with possible treatment noncompliance.

Psychiatry

History

A 26-year-old woman arrives at the emergency department by ambulance after ingesting approximately 20 pills. She apparently called emergency services shortly after taking the 50-mg amitriptyline tablets in a suicide attempt. The patient is conscious and says she wanted to "end it all." She has a history of major depression and a previous suicide attempt via acetaminophen ingestion. She denies taking any other medications, though she admits that she had "several beers" prior to taking the pills. The patient has no other past medical or psychiatric history.

Interview/Exam

T: 99.8°F   BP: 140/90   P: 98/min   RR: 16/min

The patient is mildly agitated, but alert and oriented. Her pupils are somewhat dilated bilaterally, but reactive. The chest is clear to auscultation, and no cardiac murmurs are appreciated. Pulses are strong in all four extremities. Abdominal exam is unremarkable. Reflexes are symmetric bilaterally.

The patient expresses regret at having taken the pills and says she no longer wants to die.

Tests

Hemoglobin: 14 mg/dL (normal 12–16)
Sodium: 140 meq/L (normal 135–145)
Potassium: 4.2 meq/L (normal 3.5–5)
Carbon dioxide content (CO_2): 24 meq/L (normal 24–30)
BUN: 10 mg/dL (normal 8–25)
Creatinine: 1 mg/dL (normal 0.6–1.5)
EKG: normal sinus rhythm with slight QRS prolongation (110 milliseconds)

Pathophysiology

TCA overdose is one of the **most common causes** of intentional, fatal prescription drug overdose. Incidence is slightly down due to the introduction of the less-toxic serotonin-specific reuptake inhibitors (SSRIs), but TCAs are still widely prescribed. Traditional TCAs have a **large volume of distribution** and a fairly **long half-life,** and they undergo primarily **hepatic metabolism.** They have **anticholinergic effects, alpha-blocking effects,** and **quinidine-like effects on the heart.** TCAs generally are **rapidly absorbed** from the GI tract, but active metabolites may undergo enterohepatic circulation.

Diagnosis & Treatment

Clinical effects from an overdose generally begin within the **first 6 hours after ingestion.** More than one substance may be ingested, complicating management. **Secure the ABCs** (airway, breathing, circulation) **first.**

Effects of TCA overdose include **anticholinergic signs,** such as agitation, myoclonus, mydriasis (pupils dilated), urinary retention, confusion, hallucinations, fever, hypertension, and tachycardia. With greater degrees of toxicity, **central nervous system depression, seizures, hypotension,** and **cardiotoxicity** may occur. **Cardiac arrhythmias** are one of the most feared complications of TCA overdose (and they frequently appear on USMLE exams). **QRS prolongation** (> 100 milliseconds or 0.10 seconds) is a sensitive indicator of toxicity. Tachyarrhythmias, conduction delays, and bradycardia may all occur. Avoid beta blockers and class IA antiarrhythmics (e.g., quinidine) in TCA overdose, because of the effects of TCAs on the heart.

Treatment includes establishing IV access and close monitoring of vital signs (intubate if altered mental status), EKG, and urine output, generally in an intensive care setting. **Gastric lavage followed by activated charcoal** is generally recommended if ingestion is recent (within a few hours). Give **sodium bicarbonate** to reduce cardiotoxicity in the setting of EKG changes. Give **lidocaine or phenytoin** for ventricular tachycardia, and consider cardiac pacing. Treat seizures with diazepam or phenytoin. Vasopressors and volume expansion with saline may be needed for hypotension. Death is generally a result of cardiotoxicity and/or severe hypotension.

More High-Yield Facts

Give depressed/potentially suicidal patients a prescription for only **1 week's supply** of TCA at a time (or use another drug class such as SSRIs) with **no refills** to prevent severe toxicity upon attempted overdose.

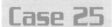

Case 25

Psychiatry

History

A 28-year-old man comes into your office at the request of his mother, though he has no complaints. His mother is worried because she says her son has no friends and never engages in social activities. She says he has never had a sexual partner or serious relationship that she is aware of and he is basically a "loner," often failing to show up even for family functions. The patient has no significant psychiatric or medical history and takes no medications. He works as a welder on the night shift and has been employed by the same company for the past 10 years. He reports no difficulties at work and denies drug or alcohol abuse.

Interview/Exam

The patient is introverted, speaks only when spoken to, and seems very uncomfortable during the interview. He is alert and oriented. He avoids eye contact and seems to have a flattened affect. The patient acknowledges his mother's comments as true and states that he has never had sexual relations, nor does he desire to have them. He seems unconcerned about his lack of friends, saying that he has never really needed them, as he obtains all the companionship he needs from his dog. His only hobby is astronomy, about which he seems to have considerable knowledge. The patient likes his job because there are few people he has to deal with on the night shift, and no one bothers him. He denies hallucinations and delusions, and his thoughts are organized and rational. He has a normal capacity for abstract thinking. Memory and concentration are normal.

Tests

None

Pathophysiology

Those with schizoid personality disorder are classic **"loners"** who enjoy living in solitude. The disorder is fairly common, and there may be a **slight male predominance.** The link or correlation between this disorder and schizophrenia does not seem to be as strong as the link between *schizotypal* personality disorder and schizophrenia. However, there is an **increased incidence of schizophrenia in first-degree relatives** of those with schizoid personality disorder.

Diagnosis & Treatment

Patients have a lifelong pattern of **social withdrawal,** with a **lack of interest in social relationships** and **restricted expression of emotions.** They often seem **isolated, quiet, distant, self-absorbed, and aloof.** Patients **neither desire nor enjoy close relationships,** including being part of a family, having friends, and having sexual partners. They almost always choose **solitary activities** and, in fact, **take pleasure in few activities.** Hobbies are generally centered around non-human interests, such as mathematics or astronomy. Patients generally show a **flattened affect, emotional coldness,** and **detachment,** and appear **indifferent to the praise or criticism of others.**

Unlike those with schizophrenia or schizotypal personality disorder, schizoid patients have **no thinking abnormalities.** They often seem somewhat eccentric, but they are **logical** and can easily recognize reality. They typically have **steady work histories,** preferring **noncompetitive jobs with minimal human contact.**

Treatment centers around **psychotherapy.** Medications may be helpful for specific symptoms.

More High-Yield Facts

People with schizoid personality disorder often **do not marry unless aggressively pursued.**

Patients with *avoidant* personality disorder are also somewhat isolated; the difference is they *desire relationships,* but avoid them because they fear rejection. Schizoid patients don't want relationships.

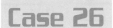

Case 26

Psychiatry

History

A 28-year-old woman requests hypnosis or whatever other treatment is available for her fear of dogs. She says she has been terrified of dogs since she was a child and has always avoided them. Recently, she met a man to whom she is attracted, but he is a dog lover and has several large dogs. She would like to overcome her fear of dogs so that she can accept an invitation over to his house for dinner.

The patient has never been attacked by a dog, and she realizes her fear of dogs is irrational. However, she describes extreme terror and difficulty breathing when around any type of dog. Her past medical and psychiatric history are unremarkable, and she takes no regular medications. She denies the use of illicit drugs and only uses alcohol on rare social occasions. The patient works as an accountant. She mentions that her mother was also afraid of dogs.

Interview/Exam

The patient is alert, oriented, and appropriate. Her affect is normal, and she does not seem depressed. Her thoughts or organized and logical, and she appears well-adjusted. You detect no abnormalities of concentration or memory during a mini-mental status evaluation. The patient denies hallucinations and delusions.

Tests

None

Pathophysiology

Phobias are the single **most common mental disorder** in the U.S., estimated to affect **5–10%** of the population, though many never seek treatment. **Females are affected twice as often** as males, and onset generally begins between childhood and early adulthood. Common specific phobias include **animals, storms, heights, blood, injections, needles, and social situations.**

Diagnosis & Treatment

Affected patients have a **marked, persistent, excessive, and unreasonable fear** that is triggered by the presence or anticipation of a **specific object or situation.** When exposed to the object or situation, patients have a **severe anxiety** response, which may take the form of a **panic attack** (e.g., terror, dizziness, difficulty breathing, palpitations, fear of dying or going crazy). Phobic patients **recognize that their fear is excessive or unreasonable,** but still **avoid the object/situation or endure it only with intense anxiety or distress.** The phobia must cause significant distress or interfere with some aspect of functioning before it is truly considered a disorder, and the fear shouldn't be due to another disorder (e.g., fear of going to school in separation anxiety disorder).

With a social phobia, people fear being exposed to **unfamiliar people or social settings** because they worry about **displaying anxiety** or doing or saying something that will **humiliate or embarrass them.** Social phobia is often considered as a separate disorder, though it is also a type of specific phobia.

Treatments generally are fairly effective for specific phobias. **Behavioral techniques** include systematic desensitization and flooding. In **systematic desensitization,** patients are told to relax and then are exposed to increasing degrees of a stimulus that resembles their phobia (e.g., think about a dog, see a drawing of a dog, hear a dog barking). In **flooding,** patients are immediately exposed to their phobic stimulus without easing into it or relaxing and are unable to escape the stimulus (e.g., locked in a room with a dog). **Hypnosis** may also be helpful in some cases. **Medications** can be beneficial, especially with social phobia. **Beta-blockers** can be used prior to exposure to the feared stimulus to reduce adrenergic symptoms. **Serotonin-specific reuptake inhibitors** and other **antidepressants** can also reduce symptoms and help prevent panic attacks upon exposure to the feared stimulus.

More High-Yield Facts

Substance abuse and depression are more common in people with phobias.

Psychiatry

History

A 58-year-old widow complains of vague abdominal pain. He has a long history of alcoholism and depression and admits to a recent increase in alcohol intake secondary to losing his job 1 week ago and the impending anniversary of his wife's death, which occurred 1 year ago. The patient's past medical and psychiatric history is significant for alcoholism, gout, depression, and a prior suicide attempt via hanging. He takes colchicine daily, but no other regular medications.

Interview/Exam

The patient is alert and oriented, but displays psychomotor retardation. You smell alcohol on his breath. Physical examination is otherwise unremarkable, with no tenderness to palpation of the abdomen, normal bowel sounds, and stool that is negative for occult blood. The patient admits to feelings of hopelessness and worthlessness and says the world would "probably be better off" without him. He apologizes for wasting your time and gets up to leave.

Tests

None

High risk for suicide

Pathophysiology

Suicide is the **9th leading cause of death** in the U.S., and the **3rd leading cause of death in adolescents.** A potential suicide is a psychiatric emergency. **Men** *commit* **suicide three times more often** than women, **but women** *attempt* **suicide four times more often.** Though the rate of suicide is **increasing most rapidly in adolescents,** suicide is most common in those **> age 45.** In general, whites commit suicide more than other races. **High social status, single/divorced/widowed** marital status, **chronic medical conditions,** history of other **psychiatric disorders, substance abuse,** age greater than 45, history of **violence or past suicidal behavior,** and **unemployment** are suicide risk factors.

Diagnosis & Treatment

It is important to **ask** about suicidal thoughts, plans, and previous attempts, especially in the setting of a depressed mood. Asking such questions does *not* increase the risk of suicide. Patients with a **specific plan** on how to carry out the suicide are considered at higher risk than those with only a vague notion of ending their life. Feelings of **hopelessness or worthlessness** are also worrisome. Self-inflicted gunshot wounds are the most common cause of death in suicide cases.

A past suicide attempt is probably the best indicator of the risk of a future suicide attempt, and the risk is highest **within 3 months** of the first attempt. **Alcohol dependence, depression, and schizophrenia** *markedly* increase the risk, but the risk of suicide is increased, to a lesser degree, by almost any psychiatric disorder.

A clinical assessment of suicide risk must be performed and a decision made about whether or not to hospitalize the patient. **High-risk patients** (as in this case) **should be hospitalized—against their will if necessary.** In determining the risk of potential suicide, age > 45, alcohol dependence, a history of violence/rage, prior suicidal behavior, and male sex are considered the **most potent risk factors** in descending order.

During hospitalization, **close supervision, psychotherapy,** and **antidepressant medications** are employed until the suicide risk has diminished enough to allow outpatient treatment.

More High-Yield Facts

Note that suicide risk is often transiently *increased* just as a patient is coming *out of* a major depression (e.g., when antidepressants begin to work). Symptoms may have improved just enough to give the patient the energy to commit suicide.

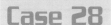

Psychiatry

History

An 18-year-old boy is brought to the emergency department by his parents after they were called by his dormitory supervisor. The supervisor told the parents that their son was displaying very unusual behavior and speech that was markedly different from when he began college 6 months earlier. The boy had become almost incoherent, using strange phrases and words that made no sense. In addition, he had been seen several times in the hallways or outside the dorm talking to imaginary people. The patient's roommate told the parents that he was "almost like a zombie," displaying little emotion and no longer attending classes. The parents state that they have been in Europe for the last 6 months on an extended business trip and are astonished at the current changes in their son.

The patient has no significant medical or psychiatric history, though the parents mention that he started to become withdrawn and express strange ideas shortly after graduation from high school. They simply thought he was going through "a phase" and were not overly concerned about his behavior at that time. He takes no regular medications and has no history of substance abuse.

Interview/Exam

The patient is alert, but disheveled appearing. His speech is disorganized and difficult to follow, at times even incoherent. During the interview, you notice the patient staring off as if listening to someone, sometimes nodding in apparent response. His affect is flat, and his reasoning concrete when it is understandable.

Tests

CT scan of the brain: negative

Pathophysiology

Schizophrenia is the classic psychotic disorder. It affects roughly **1%** of the population, both in the U.S. and most of the rest of the world, with **equal prevalence in males and females.** However, males are affected by schizophrenia about **10 years earlier** than females (peak age of onset is **15–25 in men and 25–35 in women**). Those affected are more likely to have been born in the **winter,** for currently unknown reasons. There is a **genetic component,** as the concordance rate in identical twins is nearly 50%, while a non-twin sibling of a schizophrenic has only a 10% chance of developing the disorder. Brain imaging has demonstrated **increased ventricular size** and **decreased cortical tissue volume** in affected compared to unaffected persons.

Diagnosis & Treatment

Criteria for a diagnosis of schizophrenia include **delusions, hallucinations, disorganized speech/thoughts, disorganized (or catatonic) behavior, and negative symptoms.** At least two of these criteria must be present (except in the case of bizarre delusions or hallucinations, which alone are sufficient to make the diagnosis). The diagnosis requires a total of **6 months** of symptoms, but only 1 month of active symptoms is required (i.e., may have 5 months of residual or prodromal symptoms).

With the advent of newer antipsychotics, schizophrenia treatment has focused more on the negative symptoms. These include **flattened or blunted affect, alogia (no speech), avolition (apathy), anhedonia (no pleasure), and poor attention.** Negative symptoms respond better to **atypical** (i.e., newer) **antipsychotics,** such as **risperidone** and **olanzapine,** while both atypical and traditional antipsychotics treat **positive symptoms** (e.g., hallucinations, delusions, bizarre behavior, thought disorders).

The best treatment is **antipsychotic medication plus psychotherapy / psychosocial support.** Newer antipsychotics are now **favored** due to better side-effect profiles and reduction in negative symptoms. Roughly **10–15%** of schizophrenics eventually commit **suicide.** Good prognostic features include **good premorbid functioning** (most important), **early onset, obvious precipitating factors, married, positive symptoms, good support system, and family history of mood disorders.** The opposites of these features indicate a poor prognosis (e.g., poor premorbid functioning, late onset).

More High-Yield Facts

The total **duration of symptoms** changes the diagnosis: **< 1 month** = acute psychotic disorder, **1–6 months** = schizophreniform disorder, **> 6 months** = schizophrenia.

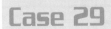

Case 29

Psychiatry

History

A 20-year-old woman has been fired from her job for repeated tardiness. She believes her tardiness is due to excessive concern over personal hygiene and she wonders if she needs help. The patient says that she washes her hands at least ten times a day, and generally re-washes them after touching any object that others may have touched first. She relates this to a concern about germs and an uncontrollable urge to keep them off her hands. The patient says that if she cannot get to a clean faucet to wash her hands quickly after an urge strikes her, she feels as though she might "explode." Several times she has had to re-wash her hands in the morning before leaving her apartment. Subsequently, she would have to stop somewhere on the way to her office, where she is a secretary, to re-wash her hands after touching a doorknob, elevator button, or other "contaminated" object. The woman knows that her excessive concerns with cleanliness and germs is unusual, but cannot prevent them from entering her mind.

The patient has no significant past medical or psychiatric history, takes no regular medications, and does not use alcohol or illicit drugs.

Interview/Exam

The patient is alert, oriented, appropriate, and intelligent. You notice that her hands are raw and erythematous, and she continuously examines them during the interview. The patient seems to become increasingly anxious, then excuses herself to go wash her hands. She seems much more relaxed when she returns. Concentration and memory are intact, and the patient denies a depressed mood or suicidal ideation.

Tests

None

Pathophysiology

OCD is estimated to affect **2–3%** of the population and has an **equal gender prevalence.** The average **age of onset is 20,** with the majority of patients having symptoms of the disorder before age 25. There is a **genetic component,** with a higher concordance rate in monozygotic twins and an increased risk in first-degree relatives. Persons with OCD have an increased incidence of **depression** (two-thirds of patients), **social phobia,** and **substance abuse.**

Diagnosis & Treatment

OCD patients have **obsessions** or **compulsions,** though **both are usually present** (at least 75% of cases). *Obsessions* are **recurrent and persistent thoughts** (or impulses) that **cause anxiety or distress** and are often experienced as **intrusive and inappropriate.** Patients recognize that these obsessions are a product of their own mind and **attempt to ignore or suppress** them, generally **without success.** The obsessions are more than just excessive worries about real-life problems; rather, they are **recognized as unreasonable, excessive, absurd, and/or irrational by those affected.**

Compulsions are **repetitive behaviors** (which may be exclusively mental behaviors, such as praying or counting) that a person **feels driven to perform,** often in response to an obsession. The goal of the behaviors is to reduce anxiety or prevent a feared event, though the behaviors are **excessive** or not realistically linked to the feared event. An obsession *increases* anxiety, while acting on a compulsion *reduces* anxiety. If a person resists carrying out a compulsion, **anxiety increases** (OCD is an anxiety disorder).

Classic obsession/compulsion pairs include **contamination/washing** or cleaning, **pathological doubt/checking** (e.g., "Did I forget to lock the door? I better go back and check." [for the 8th time]), **sexual or aggressive thoughts/confession** (e.g., confess "bad" thoughts to a priest or police officer), and the **need for symmetry/actions to create symmetry.**

The best treatment is **medications plus behavior therapy** (e.g., systematic desensitization, flooding). These therapies are probably **equally effective** when used in isolation. **Serotonin-specific reuptake inhibitors** or **clomipramine** (second choice due to side effects) are first-line medications. Approximately two-thirds of patients get better with treatment.

More High-Yield Facts

Symptoms classically begin after a **stressful life event** (i.e., death of a loved one, pregnancy), though patients may not seek treatment for years.

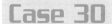

Case 30

Psychiatry

History

A 22-year-old man is seeking a referral to a surgeon who specializes in sex-change operations. He claims that he is "a woman trapped inside a man's body" and would like to "stop living a lie." The patient states that he has always felt as though he is a woman and prefers to wear women's clothes. He has changed his name from Charles to Sheila and has had electrolysis to remove his facial hair. He is wearing a dress and extensive make-up and could indeed pass for a woman based on his mannerisms and appearance. He states a sexual preference for men. The patient's past medical and psychiatric history is otherwise unremarkable, and he takes no regular medications.

Interview/Exam

The patient is alert, oriented, and intelligent. His sensorium is clear; his memory is intact; and his concentration is normal. The patient is able to reason abstractly and acts appropriately. He denies depression, but claims to be tired of living in a man's body. No hallucinations or delusions are evident.

Tests

None

Gender identity disorder (transsexualism)

Pathophysiology

Gender identity disorder is thought to be **three times more common in adult males** than females and is estimated to affect 1 in 30,000 men. Onset may occur in **early childhood,** and those affected generally experience discomfort with their genetically determined sex by **adolescence.** The cause is poorly understood, though many theories exist.

Diagnosis & Treatment

Those with gender identity disorder have a **strong and persistent identification with the opposite gender.** This is not for a cultural advantage, but rather because the person generally **feels that he or she truly is the opposite sex and was put in the "wrong body"** or feels more comfortable in the role of the opposite gender. Those who are transsexual generally wear the **clothes** of the opposite sex, **desire to live or be treated** as the opposite sex, and feel that they have the **typical feelings and reactions** of the opposite sex. They are **uncomfortable with their sex** and feel it was "inappropriately assigned." Patients generally **desire to undergo physical alterations** (e.g., **wear make-up, have electrolysis, take hormones, have a sex-change operation**) to more closely resemble the opposite sex.

In terms of reversing gender preference, treatment is **rarely successful.** In adults, treatment generally focuses on helping patients deal with the anxiety and consequences of the disorder. Sex-reassignment surgery is **controversial,** but those who desire it after psychotherapy, hormone treatment, and other options have failed to satisfy their needs are generally pleased with the results.

More High-Yield Facts

"Sex" describes the **genetic state of being male or female** and is generally determined by the **presence or absence of a Y chromosome.** Do *not* diagnose gender identity disorder in the setting of an intersex state (e.g., pseudohermaphroditism, adrenogenital syndrome, androgen insensitivity syndrome). **"Gender"** describes a **psychological state that reflects a person's sense of being male or female,** based on cultural norms.

Transvestites are **cross-dressers** (e.g., men who dress like women, daily or once a year) who are **comfortable with their sex** "assignment" and do *not* desire sexchange operations. Transsexuals and transvestites may be homosexual or heterosexual, as **sexual preference is usually unrelated to gender preference/ behavior.**

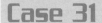

Case 31

Psychiatry

History

A 25-year-old woman presents for a follow-up visit to get test results from a work-up of her chest pain. She seems disappointed that no cause could be found for her symptoms and is not reassured by the negative results. EKG, echocardiography, CT scan, esophagogastroduodenoscopy, and multiple blood tests for autoimmune/inflammatory and infectious etiologies were all negative. Over the past 7 years, the patient has also received extensive work-ups for gastrointestinal, genitourinary, and multiple pain complaints, including headaches, low back pain, bilateral breast pain, and extremity pain and tingling—all of which posted negative results.

Interview/Exam

The patient is alert and oriented, and has a clear sensorium. She describes her chest pain in an emotional, dramatic fashion, and you note that she describes the pain differently than on the prior visit. The patient reports that she has always been sickly, which has interfered with her schooling and ability to work. She is financially independent and has never sought disability or other financial assistance. Her mood and affect are normal, and she denies depression.

Tests

See above.

Pathophysiology

Somatization is estimated to affect **1–2% of women,** and is at least **five times more common in females** than males. Some studies estimate that 5–10% of patients visiting a family or general practitioner have this disorder. It is more common in those with **little education and low income** levels, and symptoms generally begin in the **teenage years.** There is a **genetic basis** in some persons, as evidenced by twin studies and increased incidence in first-degree relatives.

Diagnosis & Treatment

Somatization disorder is characterized by **multiple physical complaints beginning before the age of 30 that occur over the course of several years and affect multiple organ systems.** The classic complaints are **pain, sexual or menstrual dysfunction,** and **gastrointestinal** and **neurological** symptoms (all should be present at some point according to DSM-IV criteria). These symptoms generally cause the patient to **seek treatment** and *cannot* be explained by physical or laboratory testing.

Complaints are often **vague,** and the history for each symptom may be **imprecise and/or inconsistent,** but *patients do not intentionally produce symptoms* (as in factitious disorder and malingering). Patients often describe their symptoms in a **dramatic, emotional, and exaggerated** fashion. They often undergo extensive testing and may have complications from invasive procedures used to diagnose or treat symptoms. Most patients believe that they have been "sickly" for most of their lives.

Regularly scheduled, brief visits to the primary care physician (e.g., once a month) should be arranged until patients can be made to realize that there may be a psychological component to their complaints and agree to see a psychiatrist. The treatment of choice is **psychotherapy,** which has been shown to reduce patients' healthcare expenditures. **Anxiety and depression** are common in affected persons and should be asked about and treated if present.

More High-Yield Facts

An association exists between **antisocial personality disorder** and somatization disorder (classic board question).

In somatization disorder, patients focus on their **symptoms,** which **change,** moving among several organ systems over time. In **hypochondriasis,** patients generally believe that they have one particular **disease,** and tend to have fairly **stable symptoms** over time.

Psychiatry

History

A 27-year-old woman comes into the office with a chief complaint of abdominal pain. She is dressed provocatively and wearing excessive make-up and jewelry. As you enter the room, you see the patient interacting with the nurse, who is male. She is openly and inappropriately flirtatious with him, and asks him to help her with her bra. When she sees you, she puts her wrist up to her forehead in an expression of exasperation and begs you to help her with the pain that has been "tormenting her forever."

Upon questioning, the patient relates a vague history of abdominal pain for the past 3 days, which she is unable to give specifics about. She suddenly begins to cry, but is quickly comforted when you tell her that you need to examine her. Your nurse returns to the room to alert you to an important phone call, and when you start to leave the room, the patient moans in pain and tells you she feels as though she may pass out. Your examination reveals no abnormalities. The patient has no significant past psychiatric history and takes no regular medications. She admits to being fairly promiscuous and is heterosexual. Chart review reveals two previous visits to your colleagues over the past 5 years for similarly vague and unimpressive complaints. There is a notation about inappropriately sexual and theatrical behavior during both visits.

Interview/Exam

The patient is alert and oriented, and has a clear sensorium. Her concentration and memory are intact, and no hallucinations or delusions are present. She is extroverted and seems to have rapidly shifting emotions. Her speech is goal-directed and not pressured; she does not seem grandiose or depressed.

Tests

None

Pathophysiology

Histrionic personality disorder affects roughly **2–3%** of the population and is **more common in females** than males. As with all personality disorders, patients have a pervasive, lifelong pattern of maladaptive traits and behaviors.

Diagnosis & Treatment

Individuals with histrionic personality disorder are **excitable, emotional, and flamboyant.** Their behavior is **colorful, dramatic, and extroverted.** The diagnosis centers on the presence of **emotionality** and **attention-seeking behavior.** Patients are **uncomfortable** when not the center of attention and classically display **inappropriate sexual, seductive, and provocative behavior.** Patients use **their physical appearance to draw attention to themselves** and display **rapidly shifting, exaggerated, and shallow emotions.** Their speech is often **impressionistic** and **lacking in detail**—dramatic flair is more important to them than accuracy and conciseness. Other signs include being **easily influenced by others** (i.e., suggestibility) and considering relationships to be more intimate than they actually are. **Somatic complaints** are common and usually vague.

Although typically sexual and provocative, patients generally are *not* sexually aggressive and often have **sexual dysfunction** (e.g., are impotent or anorgasmic). They are often described as vain and self-absorbed. When not the center of attention, patients may display temper tantrums, tears, or accusations against those around them. These individuals are fickle and are **unable to maintain deep, long-lasting relationships.**

Treatment is long-term **psychotherapy,** with adjunctive medications helpful for specific symptoms (e.g., depression, anxiety). With age, patients tend to display fewer symptoms.

More High-Yield Facts

Differentiating borderline personality disorder, narcissistic personality disorder, and histrionic personality disorder can be difficult. Those with *borderline personality disorder* are more likely to show **self-mutilating or suicidal behavior, brief psychotic episodes, and an unstable sense of self.** Those with *narcissistic personality disorder* have a **greater sense of entitlement and are more arrogant and grandiose.** The hallmark of *histrionic personality disorder* is **sexually provocative, dramatic, and theatrical behavior.**

Case 33

Psychiatry

History

A 67-year-old man has made an appointment at the request of his son. The man states that he has had great difficulty adjusting to the loss of his wife, who was killed in a car accident 3 months ago. Since her death, the patient has been in a state of shock and disbelief and has been crying on almost a daily basis. He also reports difficulty sleeping, decreased appetite, and feelings of guilt because he was supposed to have been driving his wife to her destination the day she was killed. The patient has occasionally sensed his wife's presence since she has died, though he knows these perceptions are not real, and he thought he saw her the other day at the mall before realizing the shopper was simply a woman who looks like his wife.

Interview/Exam

The patient is alert and oriented, but somewhat withdrawn. His thoughts are rational and goal-directed. He denies suicidal ideation and feelings of worthlessness and hopelessness, though he does admit to occasionally feeling that life has "lost its meaning." He describes feelings of grief coming over him in brief, sudden waves. The frequency of these feelings has decreased over the last several weeks. The patient knows that his wife is dead and will not return, but he misses her intensely. He says he has been unable to get rid of any of her personal belongings since her death, as it would be too painful for him.

Tests

None

Pathophysiology

The range of psychological reactions to a loved one's death is quite **variable,** and is influenced by **cultural norms** and the **circumstances** of the loss. For example, a sudden, unexpected death by tragic means often precipitates a more severe type of grief than an anticipated, "peaceful" death. Grief symptoms can **mimic depression** and may last for **1–2 years,** with some symptoms intermittently persisting for even longer.

Diagnosis & Treatment

"Uncomplicated" or normal grief may initially include a **state of shock,** a feeling of **numbness** or **bewilderment, intense distress, crying/sadness, sleep disturbances, decreased appetite** (may even lead to weight loss), and guilt, often called **survivor guilt.** Intense **yearning** for the deceased may occur, and some even **search for the deceased** after the death. Symptoms typically improve over time.

It is also **normal** to have **illusions** (e.g., mistaking someone's face or voice for the loved one) and even **hallucinations** (e.g., hearing the dead person's voice or feeling his/her presence), though **those with normal grief realize that these perceptions are not real.** Affected persons may refuse to discard the dead person's physical possessions in order to retain a link to the deceased. Withdrawal, apathy, and listlessness may occur once the acceptance of the person's death has begun. People may complain that "life has lost its meaning" or they are "just going through the motions."

Those with normal grief do *not* have feelings of **worthlessness** or utter hopelessness, severe **psychomotor retardation,** or **suicidal ideation.** Hallucinations or delusions about the deceased that are persistently believed to be real indicate **abnormal grief.** Persistently believing that the dead person is alive is also not normal. Note that *depressed individuals* have a **continuously depressed** mood, while *those with grief* often have intermittent **"waves"** of grief that **subside,** and they retain the ability to smile, laugh, or be happy between the periods of grief.

Treatment for normal grief/bereavement is **supportive.** *Medications are generally avoided, as they may interfere with successful resolution of the grieving process.* If abnormal grief or depression occur, psychiatric intervention is needed (e.g., psychotherapy and/or medications).

More High-Yield Facts

Normal grief is high-yield, and the boards may try to trick you into saying that a person with grief has major depression or psychosis.

Case 34

Psychiatry

History

A 24-year-old, schizophrenic man is back for a regularly scheduled visit. He seems agitated and admits that he has not been taking his medication because he doesn't like the way it makes him feel. The patient has been under your care for 6 months. When you first had contact with him it was on an inpatient basis, as he was committed involuntarily because he was severely psychotic, paranoid, and disorganized. The patient responded well to risperidone and has been doing well up until today's visit. The patient is a bus driver for a local grade school. He smokes cigarettes, but does not use alcohol or drugs.

Interview/Exam

The patient is agitated, and his speech is very disorganized. He acts extremely paranoid and makes accusations against the children he drives to school every day, saying that he will "get even" with them. He stares off intermittently during the interview, seemingly paying attention to auditory hallucinations. When you tell the patient that you are concerned about him continuing to drive the school bus while he is not taking his medications, he growls at you and runs out of the office.

Tests

None

Pathophysiology

The doctor-patient relationship is a **confidential** one. However, this confidential relationship enjoys **less protection under the law** than an attorney-client, priest-churchgoer, or husband-wife relationship. You should be aware of the exceptions to the doctor-patient confidentiality agreement and know when you need to honor it.

Diagnosis & Treatment

Exceptions to confidentiality include:
- The **patient gives you his or her permission** or asks you to reveal information. The confidentiality agreement can be broken (or waived) at **any time by the patient,** but not by the physician.
- A **court or a judge mandates you to tell** the information (this is an oversimplification, but good enough for the boards).
- Other staff members are considered to be in the "circle" of confidentiality if they are **involved in the patient's care** (e.g., the patient's nurses are privy to information, but non-participating personnel are not).
- **Suspected child abuse** (no proof needed).
- A patient is actively **dangerous to others or self.**

This last point was addressed by the famous *Tarasoff* case, which discussed the **"duty to warn"** (and protect) others or the authorities when a patient is dangerous. Classic examples of the duty to warn include:
- Patients who **threaten violence or harm to themselves or others.** In this setting, **notify the authorities** (or the individuals at risk, if appropriate) if you believe there is a definite risk of violence/harm.
- Patients with potentially life-threatening responsibilities (e.g., bus driver, airline pilot, surgeon) who show markedly **impaired judgment** (e.g., psychosis) or **physical impairment** (e.g., a patient with epilepsy who drives).

In a true emergency setting of any type, limited information should be given only to those who need it. Family members, colleagues not involved in the patient's care, the patient's attorney, and the patient's previous physician should *not* be told anything unless the patient desires it.

More High-Yield Facts

A classic board question involves your physician colleague asking about "Mrs. Smith," who you are treating, but your colleague is not. Respectfully **decline to give your colleague any information** about the patient's condition.

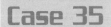

Case 35

Psychiatry

History

A 23-year-old man is brought to the emergency department by a friend because he is complaining of substernal chest pain and palpitations. The patients says that the symptoms began roughly 30 minutes ago while he was at a party. He has never experienced symptoms like this before. His past medical and psychiatric history are unremarkable.

Interview/Exam

T: 99.1°F   BP: 172/92   P: 96/min   RR: 16/min

The patient is agitated, irritable, and diaphoretic. Eye exam reveals pupillary dilatation, with a normal, symmetric reaction to light. Nasal exam reveals marked mucosal erythema and irritation, with dried blood and mucosal ulceration in the right nostril and bilateral clear rhinorrhea. No adenopathy is appreciated. The chest is clear to auscultation, and no cardiac murmurs are appreciated. The rest of the physical exam is unremarkable. During the exam, the patient becomes more agitated and begins to seem paranoid and more disorganized. He mentions that he thinks there are bugs crawling under his skin. During your mini-mental status examination, the patient has a grand mal seizure. The friend mentions that the patient may have been using drugs.

Tests

Urine drug screen: pending.
EKG: normal sinus rhythm with frequent premature ventricular complexes
CT brain scan: no abnormalities
Electrolytes: normal

Cocaine abuse

Other amphetamine or stimulant abuse is also possible.

Pathophysiology

Cocaine is a **stimulant** that **inhibits the reuptake** of catecholamines (e.g., dopamine, norepinephrine, serotonin) and also has local **anesthetic** effects. Roughly 1% of the population at least occasionally uses cocaine. Users may **snort, inject, or smoke** (freebase or crack cocaine) the drug to obtain its effects, which typically last **30–60 minutes.** Though physical addiction doesn't occur with cocaine, the **psychological addiction can be severe.**

Diagnosis & Treatment

Cocaine intoxication may result in **elation, euphoria, heightened self-esteem, increased energy, decreased appetite (and often nausea), and perceived improvement of task performance.** With higher doses, users can become **agitated, irritable, impulsive,** and physically and/or sexually **aggressive. Sympathomimetic effects** can be recognized clinically and include **mydriasis** (pupillary dilatation), **tachycardia, hypertension, psychomotor agitation, and diaphoresis.** Classic physical finding in those who use cocaine intranasally include **nasal congestion, rhinorrhea, nasal mucosal irritation and/or erythema, and nosebleeds.** Chronic users may suffer **nasal septal perforation.**

Severe intoxication can result in **vomiting, palpitations, cardiac arrhythmias, chest pain/cardiac ischemia, confusion, seizures, strokes, dyskinesias, respiratory depression, coma, and death.** Psychosis (including **formication,** or the sensation of bugs crawling under the skin, which is classic), delirium, impaired judgment, bizarre behavior, a manic-type state, severe anxiety, insomnia, and impotence may also occur.

Treatment of intoxication is **supportive.** If severe hypertension occurs, *do not use a beta-blocker,* as this can lead to unopposed alpha-stimulation and worsening hypertension. Employ a combination alpha and beta-blocker (e.g., labetalol) or another class of drug in this setting. General **addiction treatment** should be offered, using standard addiction therapy principles. Withdrawal generally causes **opposite** symptoms of intoxication: **fatigue, hypersomnia, increased appetite, depressed mood, and psychomotor retardation.**

More High-Yield Facts

Amphetamines/other stimulants generally cause symptoms **similar to cocaine,** but the half-life of these compounds is **longer.**

Smoking cocaine products can result in **lung damage** ("crack lung"), and IV use can lead to **endocarditis, HIV,** and **hepatitis B, C, and/or D.**

Case 36

Psychiatry

History

A 41-year-old man has come in for a check-up at the request of his wife. The patient says he agreed because he could "use something for sleep." The wife is concerned because her husband believes the FBI is after him and trying to ruin his life because he is a distant cousin to a deceased man who killed a police officer 15 years ago. The wife says the patient spends most of his free time looking for tangible proof of this plot against him. For example, he spends hours looking through the windows of their house with binoculars to see if FBI agents are watching him, and checking the phones for wire taps. The wife says the symptoms started gradually over the past few months, but his behavior has started to affect his work and has all but ended their social life.

The patient has no past medical or psychiatric history and takes no regular medications. His family history is noncontributory.

Interview/Exam

The patient is alert and oriented, and has a clear sensorium. His thoughts are goal-directed and organized. He seems suspicious, but is intelligent and has normal memory and concentration. He asks you if you are a member of the FBI or know anyone who works there. When you reply in the negative, the patient begins to tell you that the FBI is out to "ruin" him. He says he has heard the clicks indicating an active wire tap on his phone, though he admits that three specialty security firms he hired failed to find evidence of phone taps. He also believes his mail is being examined on a daily basis, though on the days he watches the mailman deliver the mail he has not seen this activity occur.

The patient is an accountant, with an excellent track record at work. He says he is concerned because the FBI has started to monitor him more closely in his office. He denies any criminal acts or wrongdoing and claims he is being "attacked" for what his distant cousin did 15 years ago. He believes the orders to persecute him came from the head of the FBI, who the patient knows a great deal about. The patient does not seem depressed and displays no bizarre behavior or evidence of hallucinations.

Tests

CT brain: no abnormalities

Delusional disorder

Pathophysiology

Delusional disorder is fairly uncommon, estimated to affect 1 in 3000 people. It has an average age of onset around **40 years old.** There does *not* seem to be much of a genetic component, and the etiology is unknown.

Diagnosis & Treatment

Those with delusional disorder have a **persistent delusion for more than 1 month.** The delusions are characteristically **non-bizarre** (i.e., possible, though unlikely). This is an important point to help differentiate between this disorder and **schizophrenia.** For example, a delusional patient may believe that the FBI is following him, which is highly unlikely but possible, while a schizophrenic patient may believe aliens are in control, which is considered a bizarre or impossible delusion. Other than the delusion and its impact and ramifications, patients with delusional disorder have a **normal thought process,** and **lack the bizarre behavior and severe functional impairment** seen in other psychotic disorders. Affected patients are often **employed** and may have several normal relationships.

Classic categories of delusions include: **persecutory** (**most common;** belief that one is being badly/maliciously treated in some way), **jealous** (belief that a sexual partner is unfaithful), **grandiose** (belief that one has a special power, worth, knowledge, or relationship with a famous or powerful person), and **erotomanic** (belief that another person, usually of higher status, is in love with him or her). Other types of delusions also occur, but are less common.

Treatment is **psychotherapy plus antipsychotic medications. Inpatient treatment** may be needed if violence is a concern secondary to the delusion. A general rule of thumb is that the therapist should **neither challenge nor agree with the patient's delusions initially;** rather, the therapist should focus on the **effects** the patient's delusion is having on his or her life.

More High-Yield Facts

A delusion is a **fixed, false belief** based on an **incorrect assumption** or **inference** about reality. A delusion is **inconsistent with the patient's cultural background and intelligence** and **cannot be eliminated/corrected by reasoning** (e.g., this patient's continued belief that his phones are tapped despite three security firms finding no evidence of a wire tap).

Psychiatry

History

A 34-year-old man complains of low back pain. He says he has tried every over-the-counter pain medication and several prescription medications, and none of them seem to help. The patient would like you to sign some papers so that he can go on disability, because he claims that there is no way he can perform any type of work given the severity of his pain, which is nearly constant. His past medical and psychiatric history is unremarkable, and he does not regularly take any medication. The patient claims to have had extensive work-ups with CT scan and MRI as well as "lots" of blood tests, but no one can tell him what is wrong with him.

Interview/Exam

The patient is alert and oriented, and has a clear sensorium. Several times during the interview, he winces in pain and grabs his lower back with both hands. Physical exam reveals normal neurologic responses, including normal sensation and reflexes in all extremities and a normal straight leg raise bilaterally. When you palpate the patient's lumbar spine, he dramatically winces in pain. Later in the exam, you put a similar amount of pressure on his lumbar spine while listening to his lungs, and he does not seem tender.

When you ask where to obtain copies of the patient's records, to assist in your decisions about further diagnostic steps and pain relievers, the patient becomes irritated. He agrees to send the records to you, but says, "Look doc, just sign these forms and we'll take care of that stuff on the next visit."

Tests

None

Pathophysiology

Unfortunately, malingering is fairly common, though the exact incidence is unknown. Those who malinger seek external secondary gain, and they fake symptoms of illness to acquire that gain. It is believed that **males malinger more commonly** than females.

Diagnosis & Treatment

Those who malinger **intentionally/voluntarily create symptoms** that are grossly **exaggerated,** whether **physical or psychological.** These symptoms are produced to satisfy an **external motivation.** The goal in malingering is often to **avoid difficult/dangerous situations, responsibilities, punishment, or the police;** or to **receive compensation, free room and board, or a source of drugs.** Another possible motivation is **retaliation** (e.g., for guilt, financial loss, legal penalty, job loss).

Symptoms/complaints are generally **vague,** and patients may have a fairly **savvy understanding** of the law and a standard medical work-up. Complaints such as low-back pain, headaches, neck pain, vague abdominal or chest pain, dizziness, amnesia, and anxiety are typically chosen because they are **difficult to disprove.** Patients are **more interested in compensation, avoidance of responsibility, or drugs than a cure** and may become **angry** if given a clean bill of health. In an inpatient setting, symptoms may wax and wane depending on whether or not the patient is being observed.

Certain situations should heighten your suspicion of malingering: involvement of **clear medicolegal issues** (e.g., patient referred by attorney for medical evaluation), marked **discrepancy between claimed disability and objective findings,** **lack of cooperation** during evaluation and with treatment regimen, and presence of **antisocial personality disorder.**

Treatment is difficult. Conduct a **thorough evaluation** of the patient's complaints, because malingering is often a diagnosis of exclusion. *Avoid displaying anger or suspicion.*

More High-Yield Facts

The primary difference between malingering and factitious disorder is the **patient's intent.** Patients with either disorder **intentionally create symptoms,** but the **reasons differ.** Those with factitious disorder only want to **assume the sick role/be a patient.** They seek no external (e.g., money, drugs) gain. Malingerers do *not* want to assume the sick role or be a patient; they simply use medical symptoms as a **means to an end** (e.g., to get money or drugs, avoid work).

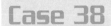

Case 38

Psychiatry

History

A 37-year-old woman is troubled by headaches and fatigue. She says that she is always tired and can't seem to sleep well, often waking up involuntarily very early in the morning. Her headaches, which she describes as dull, aching, generalized pain, are frequent. These symptoms began roughly 3 weeks ago and have been getting steadily worse. The patient also mentions a lack of interest in her hobbies, and she has missed several days of work due to fatigue. She wonders if she might have a brain tumor because she has difficulty concentrating and frequent crying spells. She also reports a loss of appetite.

The patient has no significant past medical or psychiatric history and takes no regular medications, though she has been using acetaminophen for her headaches. She denies using alcohol or drugs. The patient is married, with teenage children.

Interview/Exam

The physical examination is unremarkable. The patient is alert and oriented, and her thoughts are goal-directed and logical. During the interview, you note that she exhibits some psychomotor retardation. At one point, the patient bursts into tears. She apologizes profusely and says she has been feeling sad almost constantly lately, which she thinks may have something to do with family problems, as she has recently separated from her husband. The woman admits that she just can't seem to clear her mind of thoughts that her life is worthless. She denies current suicidal ideation.

Tests

Hemoglobin: 14 g/dl (normal 12–16)
White blood cell count: 7000/μL (normal 4500–11,000)
Basic metabolic panel: normal
Erythrocyte sedimentation rate: 8 mm/hr (normal 0–20)
Thyroid-stimulating hormone: 2.1 μU/mL (normal 0.5–5)

Major depressive disorder

The patient is experiencing a major depressive episode.

Pathophysiology

The lifetime prevalence of major depressive disorder is estimated to be **15%** overall, and **females are affected twice as often** as males. The average age of onset is 40 years old, though children and the elderly can be affected. Roughly 10% of primary care patients seen in an outpatient setting have depression. About 10–15% of affected patients commit suicide.

Diagnosis & Treatment

Depression is a common problem and should be kept in mind whenever a patient presents with **vague complaints** (e.g., headaches, abdominal pain, fatigue). Note that the patient often does not say "I'm depressed." Symptoms of depression include **depressed or sad mood** (or irritable mood in children), **loss of interest/ ability to feel pleasure** (anhedonia), **fatigue/reduced energy, lack of motivation, trouble sleeping, decreased appetite** (and possibly weight loss), **psychomotor retardation, feelings of worthlessness or inappropriate guilt, dimished ability to think or concentrate, and recurrent thoughts of death or suicide.** Withdrawal from friends, family, and activities is typical, as are loss of interest in sexual activity, **anxiety,** and **substance abuse.**

A major depressive episode is diagnosed if **multiple depressive symptoms** (at least one must be depressed mood or anhedonia) are present for **at least 2 weeks.** A single major depressive episode gives a diagnosis of major depressive disorder, unless there is a history of mania or other coexisting features that would change the diagnosis. **Recurrence** after treatment is common. Patients with severe depression may have **psychotic symptoms,** which are often **mood congruent** (i.e., have a depressed theme to them, such as death or guilt); these require treatment with antipsychotic drugs. Multiple causes of depression—including **hypothyroidism,** hypercalcemia, lupus, other medical illness (classic is pancreatic cancer), and **medications or substance abuse**—must be excluded before the diagnosis is made.

Treatment is **antidepressant medication plus psychotherapy. SSRIs** are currently favored over TCAs due to a more favorable side-effect profile. **Electroconvulsive therapy** is an option for those who fail multiple trials of medication. **Always inquire about suicidal ideation,** and hospitalize people (against their will if necessary) if the suicide risk is high.

More High-Yield Facts

Patients with *atypical* depression have *increased* **sleep and appetite/eating** (hypersomnia and hyperphagia).

Case 39

Psychiatry

History

A 28-year-old woman has come to see you because she thinks she is "going crazy." She says her symptoms started 2 months ago, roughly 2 weeks after she was raped and beaten by an unknown assailant while walking home from the grocery store near her apartment. She was hospitalized for 2 weeks due to extensive injuries and began to experience severe nightmares related to the assault a few weeks after she returned home. In addition, the patient reports severe anxiety and even panic whenever she drives past the location of the attack, which she must pass every day to get to her apartment. She states that she now shops for groceries on the other side of town and cannot even think about the name of the grocery store she used to shop at without breaking into a sweat.

The patient has been having trouble sleeping and "always feels on edge." She says the slightest things startle her now. The patient has no significant past medical or psychiatric history and takes no regular medications, though she asks if you could prescribe sleeping pills to help her sleep. She doesn't drink alcohol or use drugs. She is single and has no children.

Interview/Exam

The patient has some difficulty concentrating during the interview and seems somewhat irritable. However, she is alert and oriented and has goal-directed and coherent thoughts. She mentions a sense of detachment from her friends and family, and admits to recurrent images from the assault that seem to flash through her mind at random times, even though she tries to avoid thinking about it. The patient denies suicidal ideation, but says she wonders what her life will be like now and doubts she will ever marry.

Tests

None

Pathophysiology

PTSD describes a set of typical symptoms that occur in certain people who experience an **extremely traumatic stressor.** It has been classically described in association with combat experience (especially Vietnam), but also can occur after rape, assault, torture, natural disasters, and serious accidents. The disorder affects roughly **2%** of the general population and is most likely to occur in **younger adults** and those who are **not married, socially withdrawn,** or of low socioeconomic status.

Diagnosis & Treatment

PTSD is said to occur when people **experience a severe, often life-threatening stressor, react to the experience with fear and helplessness,** then **persistently relive the event** even though they **try not to be reminded of it or think about it.** The stressor generally is **out of the ordinary** (i.e., outside the realm of what the average person would experience). In males, a history of **combat** is classic, while **rape** is classic in females.

The re-experiencing of the event can take the form of **flashbacks, nightmares, illusions/hallucinations,** intense distress/anxiety, or somatic symptoms, which occur when the person is **exposed to cues or symbols** that are reminders of the event. Patients also **try to avoid stimuli associated with the event,** such as thoughts, conversations, activities, or places, and often report **amnesia** for at least part of the event. Patients may also experience **feeling "numb,"** detachment or estrangement from others, a restricted range of affect, and a sense of a bleak or short future (e.g., don't expect to live long, have a career, or get married). Symptoms must last at least 1 month for PTSD to be diagnosed.

Treatment includes **psychotherapy and antidepressants. SSRIs** are generally favored. **Group therapy** with others who have experienced similar trauma is often helpful, and **behavioral therapy,** such as relaxation techniques or systematic desensitization, may also be effective. PTSD patients are at increased risk of substance abuse/addiction; therefore, generally *avoid* sedatives (e.g., benzodiazepines). Note, however, that sedatives may be appropriate in *severe* cases for a *brief* period right after the stressor.

More High-Yield Facts

PTSD symptoms can begin **months or even years after** the traumatic event. The symptoms of *acute stress disorder* are **essentially identical to PTSD,** but they must begin **within 1 month** of the traumatic event and last **< 4 weeks.**

Psychiatry

History

A 19-year-old woman is brought to the emergency department because of sudden loss of vision bilaterally. Her symptoms began 4 hours ago, but she didn't tell anyone in her family for 2 hours. The patient says she is completely blind and has no light perception. She denies other symptoms, has no significant past medical or psychiatric history, and takes no medications. She denies the use of alcohol or drugs.

Interview/Exam

There are no focal neurologic deficits. The patient's pupils are normal sized, equal, and reactive to light. Funduscopic exam is normal. The patient says she is unable to count fingers and cannot see an eye chart. A nurse comes in to start an IV, and the patient withdraws her arm in fear when the nurse pulls out the needle. The remainder of the physical exam is normal.

The patient is alert and oriented, though she does not seem very concerned about her symptoms; her family members are quite concerned. The patient says her boyfriend of 2 years broke up with her last night, and she insists that he be called and told of her sudden loss of sight, as she is sure he will be very concerned and want to come to the hospital to see her.

Tests

Head CT scan: normal
Erythrocyte sedimentation rate: 9 mm/hr (normal 0–20)

Pathophysiology

Conversion disorder describes one or more neurologic symptoms that cannot be explained by a known medical disorder and are associated with identifiable psychological factors. **Females are affected at least twice as often** as males, and the disorder is most common in **adolescents and young adults.** It is typically seen in rural areas in those with **little education, low intelligence, and low socioeconomic status.**

Diagnosis & Treatment

Conversion disorder causes one or more symptoms related to a **voluntary motor or sensory function** (i.e., **neurologic symptoms**). Classic sensory symptoms are **numbness or paresthesia,** often in distributions not consistent with neurologic disease (e.g., stocking-and-glove anesthesia of the hands or feet), **blindness,** tunnel vision, and deafness. Classic motor symptoms include **weakness, paralysis, exaggerated ataxia,** and other gait problems. **Pseudoseizures** are also fairly common. **Physical findings are often inconsistent with the complaint** (e.g., normal eye exam and reaction to threatening visual stimuli in "blind" patient) or reveal symptom complexes that **can't be explained** by known disorders.

Patients also must have an **identifiable psychological conflict that is associated with or related to the symptoms.** Generally, the stressor or conflict comes right before the symptoms in an obvious **cause-effect pattern.** However, patients do *not* intentionally produce symptoms, distinguishing them from factitious disorder or malingering patients. No overt financial gain is apparent, though patients often derive **secondary gain** from the attention and support of those around them, and may exaggerate symptoms when being watched.

Symptoms generally **resolve on their own, usually within a few days,** in 90% of patients. Treatment is **brief psychotherapy.** Do *not* tell patients that they are faking their symptoms, as this can make symptoms *worse.*

More High-Yield Facts

Though not required for diagnosis, a classic finding in conversion disorder is **"la belle indifference,"** which describes an apparent **lack of concern** over seemingly serious symptoms.

Patients with **pseudoseizures** generally *do not* have incontinence, tongue biting, or injuries from falling, and pupillary and gag reflexes remain intact. A **prolactin level** drawn right after the seizure will be **normal;** in those with true seizures, it is generally **elevated.**

Psychiatry

History

A mother brings in her 15-year-old son because he has been "acting strange" lately, and she wonders if he might be depressed. She says he quit the football team, his grades have slipped over the past semester, and he often stays in his room with the door closed for several hours when he comes home from school, listening to music or sleeping. She has noticed that he cares less about his personal appearance and often seems withdrawn, suspicious, agitated, slow, and "spaced out" when he comes downstairs for dinner. The boy's eating habits have become sporadic, and she has often caught him eating ravenously late at night. The mother also notices that her son's eyes often seem red and irritated, and she wonders if he may have pink eye.

The patient has no significant past medical or psychiatric history, and he takes no regular medications. The mother doesn't think drugs are involved, but believes her son may have started smoking cigarettes, as she occasionally smells smoke on his clothes or in his room.

Interview/Exam

The patient seems annoyed and bored; he is clearly not interested in talking to you. He is of normal height, weight, and intelligence for his age, and is alert, and oriented. His thoughts are goal-directed and rational. His eyes appear normal, with no conjunctival injection appreciated. The patient is not suicidal and denies depression. He giggles when you ask him about hallucinations or delusions, but denies them. He denies drug use and says he quit football because "it's stupid," and his grades have slipped because "school is a waste of time."

Tests

None

Pathophysiology

Marijuana is by far **the most commonly used illicit drug.** Roughly 5% of U.S adults and adolescents have used it within the last month, and about 2.5% use it at least once a week. It is generally **smoked,** though it can also be eaten. Marijuana is *not* life threatening (no deaths have ever been reported) and *no* physical withdrawal syndrome is known. However, **psychological addiction and cravings can be severe,** and **tolerance** to the effects may develop. Marijuana is *not* a proven teratogen.

Diagnosis & Treatment

The symptoms of marijuana intoxication include **disinhibition, euphoria, anxiety, agitation, withdrawal, suspiciousness, paranoia, and/or temporal distortion** (person often feels that time is going very slowly and thoughts are occurring rapidly). **Impaired judgment, attention, and reaction time** (people often seem slow) may occur, as may **illusions, depersonalization, and derealization** (and, rarely, hallucinations). Classic signs of marijuana use are **conjunctival injection, increased appetite** ("the munchies"), **dry mouth, and tachycardia.**

Apathy and a lack of motivation (**amotivational syndrome**) are classic associations with chronic marijuana use. Long-term use can lead to similar health problems as cigarette smoking, such as **chronic obstructive pulmonary disease and lung cancer.**

After smoking marijuana, the peak effect usually occurs **within 30 minutes** and lasts 2–4 hours, though some impairment in motor and cognitive functions may persist for **up to 12 hours.** Marijuana as a therapeutic agent is controversial to **treat nausea** in cancer and AIDS patients. **Dronabinol,** a synthetic form of the active ingredient in marijuana (THC), is used for this exact purpose.

Treatment for chronic abuse involves counseling and standard addiction therapy (i.e., abstinence and support).

More High-Yield Facts

Marijuana intoxication can produce psychosis, delirium, and severe anxiety/panic attacks, though these effects are rare.

Marijuana can be detected in the urine for **up to 4 weeks** after the last use.

Psychiatry

History

A 34-year-old man pays you a visit with his wife of 10 years. The patient's wife says that she cannot tolerate her husband's behavior any longer and that coming to see you is a last-ditch effort to save their marriage. The woman says that her husband is constantly accusing her of infidelity with every adult figure in their lives, though she has never been unfaithful or given him any reason to worry. She also says that her husband is constantly complaining about coworkers who are "out to get him" and a boss that is plotting to have him fired, yet they are all nice people who speak highly of her husband's work. In addition, she states that her husband is suspicious of everyone he meets and bears tremendous grudges against several neighbors for minor incidents that have occurred over the years. The patient has apparently sued three different neighbors for things such as violations of the building code and failing to maintain their property. The wife is afraid to invite people over, as her husband will almost invariably misinterpret other people's friendly remarks as insults and react angrily and with excessive hostility.

The patient has no significant medical or psychiatric history. The wife claims that the symptoms she has described have been present to some degree since she first met him. He takes no medications and does not drink alcohol or use drugs.

Interview/Exam

The patient is alert and oriented. His demeanor is serious, and he seems hostile, irritable, and defensive. His thoughts are logical and goal-directed. He does not think he has a problem and does not desire treatment. When asked about his wife's comments, the patient claims that his wife is naïve and doesn't understand how things work in the real world. He admits to conflicts at work and with the neighbors and that he suspects his wife is having an affair. He feels that his coworkers gang up on him because he works harder than they do, and the neighbors are jealous because his yard is better maintained than theirs. The patient denies depression, hallucinations, and delusions.

Tests

None

Pathophysiology

Paranoid personality disorder is estimated to affect **1–2%** of the population and is **more common in males** than females. **Minority groups and immigrants** are thought to be more commonly affected than other groups. There may be some genetic basis for the disorder, as relatives of those with schizophrenia have a **higher incidence** of paranoid personality disorder.

Diagnosis & Treatment

Individuals with paranoid personality disorder have a **constant distrust and suspiciousness of others** that pervades all aspects of their lives. Affected patients interpret the actions of others as **demeaning or threatening,** and suspect (without proof or a reasonable basis) that **others are out to exploit, harm, or deceive them.** They **doubt** the loyalty and trustworthiness of friends and associates; thus they are **reluctant to confide in others** and often **read hidden or threatening meanings** into friendly or benign remarks or events. In addition, patients often **bear grudges, perceive attacks on their character or reputation** (and are quick to react angrily or counterattack), and (classically) **question their spouse's fidelity** without justification.

Classic presentations are the **bigot,** the **pathologically jealous spouse,** and the person who **frequently sues other people.** Patients have the classic defense mechanism of **projection,** where their own unacceptable impulses and thoughts are attributed to others. Patients are generally **serious** and **unable to relax,** and appear to be **unemotional.** Notably *absent* are psychotic features, fixed delusions, and overly emotional behavior.

Treatment is **psychotherapy,** though patients rarely seek psychiatric help on their own. Adjunctive medications to treat agitation may be needed.

More High-Yield Facts

Though patients always seem to be paranoid, their thoughts are generally **logical,** and they *don't* have fixed delusions. For example, a patient may believe that his spouse is having an affair, but if shown sufficient proof that he is wrong, the belief will **go away** (at least temporarily). The delusional individual will **continue to have a belief even after being shown sufficient proof that the belief is false.**

Psychiatry

History

A 34-year-old woman is brought to the emergency department by the police, who found her wearing only an open bathrobe and walking aimlessly through a nearby park. The woman claims to be the goddess of fertility; you are able to discern this though her speech is often difficult to understand. She has a long history of admissions for both manic and depressive symptoms, and was also admitted twice in the last year for severe psychosis without any apparent mood disturbance. The patient's last admission was 2 weeks ago for severely paranoid delusions, also without evidence of a mood disturbance. She escaped from custody 3 days ago just as her psychotic symptoms were starting to become controlled. She is not taking any medications currently and denies the use of drugs or alcohol.

Interview/Exam

The patient alternates between euphoria and irritability. Her speech is circumstantial and rapid. Her thoughts are disorganized and often incoherent. She continues to insist that she is the goddess of fertility and waves her arms in the air in a bizarre fashion. The patient says she has not slept in 2 days.

Tests

None

Pathophysiology

As the name implies, patients with schizoaffective disorder have symptoms of both **schizophrenia** and an **affective (mood) disorder.** Less than 1% of the population is estimated to be affected. The first-degree relatives of affected patients have an **increased incidence of mood disorders and schizophrenia,** suggesting a possible genetic component.

Diagnosis & Treatment

The key to the diagnosis is that patients must have at least **one uninterrupted period of illness during which an episode of mania or major depression occurs, and the episode must be either preceded or followed by a 2-week period of delusions or hallucinations without the presence of mood symptoms.** The mood symptoms generally predominate over the psychotic symptoms during the course of the illness, which is chronic. Patients may have only manic episodes, only depressed episodes, or both.

Treatment involves **separate therapy** for the mood component and the psychotic component. Those with manic symptoms are generally given a **mood stabilizer,** while those who only have depressive symptoms are given an **antidepressant medication** (or other depression treatment, such as electroconvulsive therapy if medications fail). Typically, **antipsychotics** are needed only briefly because the mood symptoms dominate the clinical picture. **Simultaneous use of antipsychotic and mood stabilizer/antidepressant medications may be necessary.**

The prognosis for schizoaffective patients is better than for schizophrenic patients, but worse than for those with only a mood disorder.

More High-Yield Facts

The differentiation between a **mood disorder with psychotic features** and schizoaffective disorder can be **difficult,** especially on initial/acute presentation. Those with psychosis may need to be stabilized with an antipsychotic before mood symptoms can be recognized. The key to the diagnosis of schizoaffective disorder is that at least a 2-week period of pure psychotic symptoms (without mood symptoms) must occur, which does *not* happen in those with a mood disorder that has psychotic features (because **treatment of the mood disorder makes the psychosis go away**).

Psychiatry

History

You are called to evaluate whether or not a patient is competent to make his own medical decisions. The patient's changed mental status after hospital admission has prompted his surgeon to wonder whether or not the patient is able to give informed consent for a procedure deemed medically necessary. The patient is a 62-year-old, successful attorney who was admitted for severe community-acquired pneumonia and started on intravenous antibiotics and fluids the previous night. His past medical history is notable for diabetes and hypertension, and he takes metoprolol and metformin. He has no history of psychiatric problems and has no known history of alcohol or drug abuse.

Interview/Exam

T: 103.2°F   BP: 110/70   P: 108/min   RR: 18/min   Pulse oximetry: 86%

The patient is diaphoretic and tachypneic. He is alert and knows his name, but is agitated and confused, thinking he is at home in his bedroom and that it is the year 1999. He is unable to give full attention to you and your questions, being easily distracted by other stimuli. He cannot perform serial sevens or remember three named objects 5 minutes after being told to remember them.

You speak with the patient's nurse, who states that the patient was carrying on a conversation with his wife 20 minutes ago, though the wife wasn't in the room. The nurse indicates that the patient was pleasant, oriented, and coherent when he was admitted last night.

Tests

Multiple labs pending

Pathophysiology

Delirium is **extremely common in a hospital setting,** and is thought to affect approximately 15% of patients on a general medical or surgical ward at some point during their hospital stay. The percentage becomes much higher for sicker, critical care patients (**"ICU psychosis"**). Delirium is more common in the **elderly,** those with **previous brain damage** (e.g., Alzheimer's disease, stroke), and those with **alcohol dependence.**

Diagnosis & Treatment

Delirium characteristically has an **acute onset** and a **fluctuating course.** Patients can have all of the symptoms of dementia, including **impaired memory, thinking, and judgment,** as well as **disorientation and hallucinations.** Symptoms may get worse at night (**"sundowning"**), which can also happen with dementia.

The global clouding of consciousness or **decreased consciousness is fairly unique to delirium, as persons with dementia are usually alert.** A history of a precipitating medical condition is also common in delirious patients, though the sensory deprivation and disorientation that are experienced in the critical care wards of many hospitals are often enough to cause delirium in and of themselves in many patients.

There are many medical problems to consider when someone becomes delirious, but the common ones are **hypoxia, electrolyte imbalances, infection,** renal or hepatic failure, medication reactions, hypoglycemia, endocrine dysfunction, and **substance abuse or withdrawal.** A delirious patient is **incompetent** *while he or she is delirious,* but may become competent in between episodes of delirium. Delirium can be **superimposed** on dementia, which is a diagnosis that often can only be made if the history of dementia is known.

More High-Yield Facts

Classic differential points:

	Delirium	*Dementia*
Onset	Acute & dramatic	Chronic & insidious
Common Causes	Illness, toxin, withdrawal	Alzheimers', multi-infarct dementia, HIV/AIDS
Reversible	Usually	Usually not
Attention	Poor	Usually unaffected
Arousal Level	Fluctuates	Normal

Psychiatry

History

A 27-year-old woman is brought to the office by her ex-husband with a chief complaint of being afraid to leave the house. The patient says she would have been unable to come see you today if her ex-husband had not accompanied her. She explains that she has had two episodes of severe chest pain with associated palpitations, shortness of breath, and dizziness over the last 3 months. During these episodes the woman felt as though she was dying. Extensive cardiac, respiratory, endocrine, infectious, and metabolic work-up has not revealed the cause of her symptoms. The patient is afraid to leave the house alone or be in a confined or crowded area because she fears she may have another one of these "attacks."

Over the last 6 weeks, the woman has only left the house to go to work, and has even had her groceries and other needed items delivered to avoid having to go outside. The patient has no past medical or psychiatric history, takes no medications, does not use drugs or alcohol, and is currently single, having divorced her husband 1 year ago.

Interview/Exam

The patient is somewhat anxious, but is alert, oriented, and intelligent. Her thoughts are logical and goal-directed. She denies depression or suicidal ideation. Her memory, concentration, and judgment are normal, and her affect is appropriate. The patient acknowledges that her fear of having another attack has profoundly changed her normal daily routine, and she wonders if she might be going crazy. She says that she wishes the doctors would hurry up and find out what is wrong with her so she can get on with her life.

Tests

See above.

Pathophysiology

Panic disorder with agoraphobia is a fairly **common** disorder, affecting roughly 2–4% of the population. **Females are affected two to three times more often** than males. Most patients have at least one other psychiatric disorder, such as **depression,** other **anxiety disorders, personality disorders, or substance abuse–related disorders.**

Diagnosis & Treatment

A panic disorder is diagnosed when **recurrent ($\geq$ 2) panic attacks** occur, and one of the attacks is followed by at least **1 month of worry about having another attack,** concern about an attack's consequences, and significant **behavioral changes.** Agoraphobia occurs in about **half** of those with panic disorder, and *rarely* occurs in the absence of panic attacks.

Agoraphobia describes **anxiety about being in places or situations from which escape might be difficult or embarrassing or in which help may not be available.** This anxiety is related to the person's **fear of having a panic attack** while in these situations or places. Classic specific descriptions of this fear include **fear of leaving the house, being in a crowd,** standing in a line, being on a bridge, and/or **riding in a bus, train, or automobile.** Patients will **avoid** these activities completely, endure them with great anxiety/distress, or **require the presence of a companion** to endure them.

Treatment is **psychotherapy,** often with behavioral and relaxation techniques, plus **antidepressants or anxiolytics. SSRIs** are generally preferred due to their favorable side-effect profile. Sedating anxiolytics such as alprazolam (i.e., benzodiazepines) are usually *avoided* for long-term treatment due to concerns over side effects and the potential for abuse/dependence, but are **immediately effective,** while SSRIs/other antidepressants require at least a few weeks to work in most cases.

More High-Yield Facts

Symptoms of a panic attack can mimic serious medical conditions, which **must first be excluded.** The presentation of a panic attack may closely resemble a myocardial infarction, arrhythmia, pulmonary embolus, drug intoxication/withdrawal, asthma, hypoglycemia, or pheochromocytoma. However, patients having a panic attack are generally **young and otherwise healthy,** and symptoms generally **resolve on their own within 30 minutes.**

Psychiatry

History

A 37-year-old man complains of headaches, irritability, and fatigue. He says his symptoms only occur on Saturday and Sunday, which is very annoying because he works during the week and has weekends off. He almost invariably begins to experience fatigue; throbbing, generalized headaches; irritability; and waning concentration by Saturday afternoon and doesn't feel normal again until mid-morning Monday.

The patient is married with two children and says he has no family troubles. He has no significant past medical or psychiatric history and takes no regular medications. The patient does mention drinking 8–10 cups of coffee per day at work so that he can stay focused. He doesn't drink coffee on the weekends. The patient denies illicit drug use and drinks alcohol only on rare social occasions.

Interview/Exam

Vital signs and physical examination are unremarkable. The patient is alert and oriented, with appropriate affect. He does not appear depressed, and his thoughts are clear and logical. Intelligence, memory, and concentration all seem normal.

Tests

None

Pathophysiology

Caffeine is a member of the **methylxanthine** class of agents (which includes **theophylline**) and works by **inhibiting phosphodiesterase,** which increases intracellular cyclic-AMP. Other mechanisms, such as adenosine antagonism, may be responsible for the effects of caffeine on the central nervous system. Caffeine is consumed regularly by **over 80%** of U.S. adults and has a half-life of roughly **5 hours.** Effects include **increased alertness,** a sense of well being, improved verbal and motor performance, **diuresis, cardiac muscle stimulation, increased peristalsis, increased gastric acid secretion, and increased blood pressure.** **Tolerance** to the effects of caffeine does develop, and signs of **physical withdrawal** may occur.

Diagnosis & Treatment

Caffeine intoxication can cause the above symptoms/signs plus **nervousness, restlessness, excitement, insomnia, flushed face, gastrointestinal complaints, muscle twitching, rambling speech, tachycardia, and psychomotor agitation.** Cardiac arrhythmias, tinnitus, and flashes of light may occur in some patients. With doses greater than 10 grams, **seizures, respiratory failure, and death** may occur (the average cup of coffee has roughly 100 mg of caffeine).

The classic withdrawal signs are **fatigue, headaches, irritability, and trouble concentrating. Craving** for caffeine is also common. Nausea, impaired psychomotor performance, and even anhedonia or depression can occur in some cases. Withdrawal symptoms begin **within 24 hours** and generally peak within 48 hours.

Treatment is **abstinence.** Acetaminophen or aspirin can be used until headaches resolve. Withdrawal usually takes **4 or 5 days** and is *not* dangerous.

More High-Yield Facts

Elimination of caffeine may help **peptic ulcers heal, reduce gastroesophageal reflux symptoms,** and reduce the symptoms of **fibrocystic breast disease** in some women.

Caffeine can be found in tea, many sodas, cocoa, chocolate, and many over-the-counter cold preparations, and is an effective component of some prescription preparations for **migraine** headache.

Psychiatry

History

A 27-year-old advertising executive has made an appointment at the request of his girlfriend because of "mood swings." The patient doesn't think he has a problem, but knows that he has "good days" and "bad days." He has experienced episodes of feeling "down" for 2–3 weeks at a time over the last 5–6 years. During these episodes, he becomes unmotivated, stays in bed 12–14 hours a day, and often neglects responsibilities. The patient also has periods of feeling "really good," with a markedly decreased need for sleep and increased productivity at work. He says that some of his best ideas for work projects come while he feels this way, but he also gets into trouble because he tends to be promiscuous during these periods. The patient states that he rarely goes for more than a week without being in either a "good period" or "bad period." Currently, he is feeling "pretty normal."

The patient has no other significant psychiatric or medical history and does not use drugs. However, he often drinks alcohol during the "good" days while at the numerous social functions he attends during these periods, and he believes it helps him fall asleep. He takes no medications. His father has "manic-depression."

Interview/Exam

Vital signs and physical examination are unremarkable. The patient is alert and oriented, with appropriate affect. He denies feeling depressed or having suicidal ideation, and his thoughts are clear and logical. The patient seems to have normal intelligence, memory, and concentration.

Tests

None

Pathophysiology

Cyclothymia is essentially a mild form of **bipolar disorder. Females are affected slightly more often** than males, and most patients have an onset of symptoms between **15 and 25 years** of age. Roughly 30% of patients have a **positive family history for bipolar disorder.** Relatives of those with bipolar disorder have an increased risk of cyclothymic disorder, supporting a possible genetic basis.

Diagnosis & Treatment

For at least **2 years,** affected patients have **numerous episodes of hypomania** and of **depressive symptoms,** but never meet the criteria for full-blown mania or a major depressive episode. During the 2-year period, patients never go for more than **2 months at a time** without having symptoms. Essentially, the main difference between the hypomania and the depressive symptoms in cyclothymic disorder and true mania or major depression is the **absence of functional impairment or significant distress** due to the symptoms.

Cyclothymic patients tend to have **more frequent "cycling,"** or shifting from depressive to hypomanic symptoms, than those with bipolar disorder. Patients with cyclothymic disorder are *not* severely impaired, are *not* psychotic, and do *not* generally require hospitalization. However, about **one-third** of patients will eventually go on to develop major depression or mania at some point (changing their diagnosis).

The cornerstone of treatment is **mood stabilizers,** such as **valproic acid** or **lithium. Antidepressants must be used with caution** in cyclothymic patients, as they have a markedly increased risk of **antidepressant-induced hypomanic or manic episodes.**

More High-Yield Facts

Bipolar II disorder is similar to cyclothymic disorder, but patients have episodes of **hypomania** alternating with true, full-blown episodes of **major depression** (not just depressive symptoms, as in cyclothymia).

Rule out **substance abuse,** which can cause frequent mood swings. As with almost all mood disorders, patients with cyclothymia are at **increased risk of substance abuse.** Some attribute this to patients trying to self-medicate their mood disorder.

Psychiatry

History

A 32-year-old man is in for a follow-up visit after having an MRI of the brain last week. He initially presented for frequent headaches and dizziness of 12-week duration and was convinced that he had a brain tumor, though his exam revealed no neurologic deficits. Four weeks ago, the patient had a negative CT scan of the brain and a negative lumbar puncture, but he was not convinced that he was healthy and requested that an MRI be performed. When he was told that the MRI was probably unnecessary, he insisted that one be performed and paid for the scan out of his own pocket. The patient is very anxious about the results and called your office several times during the week to see if they were available.

You inform the patient that the MRI was negative. He does not seem reassured and asks about a possible PET scan, which he read about last night on the internet. When asked why he thinks he has a brain tumor, the patient says he doesn't know and that maybe his worries are needless, but yet he asks you again about the feasibility of scheduling him for a PET scan. The patient is an accountant, is married, and does not take any regular medications or use drugs or alcohol.

Interview/Exam

The physical examination, including a thorough neurologic evaluation, are unremarkable. The man is anxious, but is alert and oriented. He denies feeling depressed or having suicidal ideation. His sensorium is clear, his thoughts are organized, and he appears to have above-average intelligence. He denies relationship or work difficulties, though he admits to frequently thinking about the possibility that he may have a brain tumor.

Tests

Electrolytes: normal
Thyroid-stimulating hormone: 2.3 μU/mL (normal 0.5–5)
Erythrocyte sedimentation rate: 9 mm/hr (normal 0–20)

Pathophysiology

Hypochondriasis is a somatoform disorder believed to be present in **5–10% of patients** in a general medical practice. It seems to affect men and women with equal frequency. Almost any age group can be affected, but the peak incidence of the disorder is in those aged **30–50.** There may be an increased familial incidence.

Diagnosis & Treatment

Hypochondriasis describes an **excessive concern about or fear of having a disease** and a **preoccupation with one's health.** This fear **persists despite medical assurance** and negative work-up. In hypochondriasis, patients interpret their symptoms or signs as evidence of physical illness. The most common complaints are pain and gastrointestinal and cardiovascular symptoms. Patients with hypochondriasis **believe that they have a serious disease that has not been detected yet** and cannot be persuaded that they don't have the disease. The belief is not of a delusional intensity, but is persistent.

A full medical work-up of the symptoms must be undertaken, as this is a **diagnosis of exclusion.** Symptoms are *not* intentionally produced, as in factitious disorder and malingering. This disorder can be differentiated from **somatization disorder** because patients with hypochondriasis focus on a **disease,** while those with somatization disorder focus on **multiple different symptoms** without focusing on what disease is causing them. In practice, this can be a difficult differential.

In hypochondriasis, patients are usually **resistant to psychiatric treatment,** as they don't believe they have a psychiatric disorder. Some may agree to "stress reduction" sessions, which can often be effective, especially in a group setting. The cornerstone of management is **frequent, regularly scheduled visits and physical examinations** to **reassure** the patient and let him or her know that the **complaints are being taken seriously.** Prognosis is **variable,** with roughly two-thirds of those affected having a chronic, waxing and waning course, and another 20% doing poorly.

More High-Yield Facts

Coexisting **anxiety and/or depression are common,** and should be asked about and treated if present.

Don't accuse patients with this disorder of faking symptoms. However, ask if stress might play some role in making symptoms worse or harder to deal with.

Psychiatry

History

A 30-year-old man states that he needs to "find out what is wrong with me." The patient says he is a perfectionist and a "workaholic," and that these traits have caused him a great deal of trouble at work and in his social life. He is an architect, and he is often criticized for missing deadlines because he is constantly "tinkering" with his work to make it better. He has had projects approved in the past, but refused to submit them to his client because he didn't feel the work met his own personal standards of excellence. The patient speaks of the importance of having a certain way of doing things and following the standards and rules set by his company. He admits to frequent frustration with his coworkers for their constant desire to "turn things upside down" by making policy changes and for their lack of adherence to company policies, such as the dress code and punctuality. He is afraid to delegate any of his work to people who "don't seem to care about order and discipline"; therefore, he has to work longer hours.

The patient says he works 7 days a week, generally at least 10 hours a day, and hasn't taken a vacation in 5 years. He has no debts and admits that he has great difficulty parting with his money. The patient hasn't been on a date or had a girlfriend in 10 years and admits to having very few friends. He would like to have more friends, but feels that most of the people he meets have loose morals and a lack of values. The patient has no significant past medical or psychiatric history, takes no medications, and doesn't drink alcohol or use illicit drugs.

Interview/Exam

The patient has a very formal, somewhat rigid demeanor. When asked open-ended questions, he seems to have a very hard time deciding how to answer. He is alert and oriented and has a clear sensorium, organized thoughts, and normal concentration and memory. His affect seems somewhat restricted, and the patient admits that he almost never feels sentimental or affectionate. He also seems to lack a sense of humor.

Tests

None

Pathophysiology

Obsessive-compulsive personality disorder is **more common in men** than women and is more often seen in **oldest children.** There is an **increased risk** of this disorder in the first-degree relatives of those who are affected. This disorder should not be confused with obsessive-compulsive disorder, which is an *anxiety* disorder, not a *personality* disorder.

Diagnosis & Treatment

Patients with obsessive-compulsive personality disorder have a pervasive pattern of **inflexibility and perfectionism,** which often interferes with task completion. They are **preoccupied with regulations/rules, details, neatness, and orderliness**—to the extent that the major point of the activity is lost. **Excessive devotion to work** and productivity preclude patients from enjoying leisure activities and friendships. Patients are also **cheap, indecisive** (due to fear of making mistakes), **overconscientious, inflexible with regard to morals/ethics/values, and overly serious.** They have a **restricted expression of affection, lack spontaneity,** and have a poor sense of humor. Affected persons **strongly dislike change** and do poorly in situations/occupations that involve flexibility, creative thinking, and shifting responsibilities.

Treatment is **psychotherapy.** Unlike most patients with personality disorders, those with obsessive-compulsive personality disorder **often seek treatment on their own** and know that they are suffering. Treatment is difficult and requires a long-term commitment. **Group and behavioral therapy** may help force patients to develop new coping strategies. **Depression** commonly develops in these patients at some point and may require medications.

More High-Yield Facts

Obsessive-compulsive disorder (OCD) is characterized by recurrent, specific **obsessions** (thoughts) and **compulsions** (behaviors), which are generally *absent* in those with obsessive-compulsive personality disorder. Some of those with the personality disorder may eventually develop OCD.

Patients often have a childhood characterized by **harsh discipline.**

Many patients with this disorder get married and hold steady jobs, though they almost invariably have **few friends.**

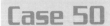

Psychiatry

History

A 72-year-old woman is brought to the office by her daughter, because the daughter is concerned that mom may have Alzheimer's disease. The patient has been complaining of memory loss and forgetfulness, which began 4 weeks ago and have rapidly worsened. Before this time, she was of sound mind and had a very good memory. The patient also complains of difficulty concentrating, indecisiveness, and trouble sleeping. The daughter states that her mother seems to have lost interest in her friends and hobbies. The patient has no significant past medical or psychiatric history and takes only acetaminophen regularly for osteoarthritis. She does not drink alcohol or use illicit drugs.

Interview/Exam

Vital signs and physical exam are normal. The patient responds to many basic questions by saying "I don't know" or "I can't remember." She has obvious psychomotor retardation. The patient does not know what year it is, but at one point in the conversation makes a reference to a recent law that was passed by the state senate. Her attention and concentration seem normal, but her task performance is inconsistent. The woman cries at one point during the interview, saying her mind "is gone."

Tests

Hemoglobin: 13 g/dL (normal 12–16)
Complete metabolic panel: normal
Thyroid-stimulating hormone: 2.3 μU/mL (normal 0.5–5)
Erythrocyte sedimentation rate: 6 mm/hr (normal 0–20)
MRI of the brain: normal
Lumbar puncture: normal
Vitamin B12 level: normal
VDRL syphilis test: normal

Pathophysiology

Pseudodementia describes **cognitive dysfunction** (i.e., dementia-type symptoms) **that occurs as a result of depression.** When the depression is treated successfully, the cognitive dysfunction goes away. This disorder classically occurs in the elderly (15% of **elderly** depressed patients present with pseudodementia), though severe depression at almost any age can cause pseudodementia-type symptoms.

Diagnosis & Treatment

Depression may cause patients to have **memory problems and cognitive loss.** However, several key points help differentiate pseudodementia from dementia. In pseudodementia, symptoms often **progress rapidly** (over the course of days or weeks) and medical attention is sought **early in the course,** while Alzheimer's dementia has an **insidious onset** over years that is often **not recognized** by the patient or their family until fairly advanced. Patients and family are both painfully **aware of the cognitive dysfunction** in pseudodementia and can often state the date when it began

With true dementia, patients generally try to **conceal their disability,** while those with pseudodementia usually **complain in detail about their cognitive deficits.** Attention and concentration are generally **preserved** in pseudodementia, but lost in dementia. Patients with pseudodementia often answer **"I don't know"** or "I can't remember." Those with true dementia try to **hide their loss of memory** and may change the subject, give vague answers, or angrily refuse to answer the question. Task impairment (e.g., serial 7's) is **variable** in pseudodementia and **consistent** in true dementia. Lastly, patients with pseudodementia often display the **symptoms of depression** (e.g., crying spells, sleeping difficulty, lack of appetite, psychomotor retardation, loss of interest in activities) and may have a history of depression.

Treatment is **antidepressant medications** (e.g., SSRIs) and **psychotherapy.** In pseudodementia, the cognitive deficits **resolve** once the depression is effectively treated. Those with dementia can become depressed, and the depression should be treated in this situation as well. The history will generally help you distinguish these two. In difficult cases, **always treat the depression** to see if the cognitive deficits improve.

More High-Yield Facts

A recent life stressor may **trigger** an episode of depression, so be alert for mention of a trigger on the boards.

CASE INDEX

Notes

Notes

Notes

Notes

Notes

Notes

Notes

Notes

Notes

Notes

Notes

Notes

Notes

Notes

Notes

Notes

Notes

Notes

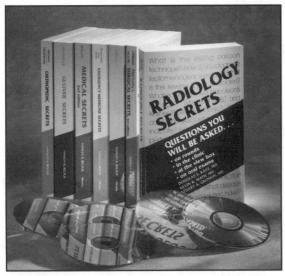

More Board Review Help

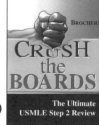
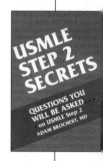
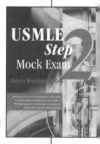
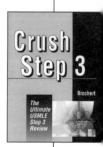